Stewart Clark

Practical Observations on the Hygiene of the Army in India

Including Remarks on the Ventilation and Conservancy of Indian prisons

Stewart Clark

Practical Observations on the Hygiene of the Army in India
Including Remarks on the Ventilation and Conservancy of Indian prisons

ISBN/EAN: 9783337126469

Printed in Europe, USA, Canada, Australia, Japan

Cover: Foto ©ninafisch / pixelio.de

More available books at **www.hansebooks.com**

PRACTICAL OBSERVATIONS

ON THE

HYGIENE OF THE ARMY IN INDIA:

INCLUDING REMARKS ON THE

VENTILATION AND CONSERVANCY OF INDIAN PRISONS;

WITH A CHAPTER ON PRISON MANAGEMENT.

ILLUSTRATED WITH WOODCUTS.

BY STEWART CLARK, M.R.C.S. ENG.,

INSPECTOR-GENERAL OF PRISONS, NORTH-WEST PROVINCES, INDIA.

LONDON:

SMITH, ELDER, AND CO., 65, CORNHILL.

1864.

PREFACE.

The sanitary condition of the British Army in India has of late been the subject of anxious inquiry. It is hoped that the practical suggestions made in this treatise may prove of use at the present time.

It has not been my object to enter into any elaborate discussion on the composition of foul air and impure water. Our knowledge of these, particularly the former, is, in some respects, involved in considerable obscurity; and many of the arguments relating to the gases, vapours, and other substances in which are supposed to lie their peculiar poisonous qualities, are purely hypothetical. But, however various the opinions regarding the particular gases or vapours in impure air which generate certain diseases, and however difficult it may be to exactly define its true character, all are agreed as to its generally baneful influence on the human constitution, and the healthful, invigorating effect of living in a pure atmosphere.

The out-door labourer, who works from morning till night in the open air, endures for years a great amount of toil, often on poor fare, and indifferently housed at night, yet all the while is strong and in robust health. The hardy Scotch Highlander is able to walk forty, fifty, and even sixty miles a day among his native hills, on no better fare than a dish of porridge and a piece of oatmeal cake; and this chiefly in consequence of the pure air in which the greater part of his life has been passed. So also, the Indian palanquin-bearer, who lives much in the open air, and has never more than two meals a day (and often not more than one), consisting of chupattes and a little ghee,* will endure the toil of carrying a heavy load twenty-five, thirty, and even thirty-five miles a day continuously, without over-fatigue, and seldom ailing.

But the difference in the same classes of men is remarkable when they are congregated in ill-ventiated workshops and barracks, although they live at the same time on the best food that can be procured. The artisan soon loses his healthy, robust appearance, becomes sickly, and dies at an early age; and the soldier, who in times of peace lives, to all appearance, in comfortable quarters and is fed sumptuously, is easily fatigued, hardly able to endure a march of ten

* Unleavened cakes and clarified butter.

or fifteen miles, is often sickly, and falls a ready prey to cholera or any other passing epidemic.

Whenever any epidemic or contagious disease prevails in any group of individuals or locality, to such an extent as to call for an inquiry into the probable cause of it, whatever other causes may be advanced to account for the calamity, we are sure to find want of proper ventilation or the presence of foul air in some shape prominent amongst them. From one source and another we have sufficient evidence to prove that many of the worst evils to which human flesh is heir, originate in the inhalation of impure air, rendered so by animal effluvia; hence our best exertions should be used to render the air of the apartments and localities inhabited by us, and by those of whom we have responsible charge, as pure as possible.

In a paper read before the British Association for the Advancement of Science, in August, 1863, I submitted a few observations on the baneful effects of foul air, and offered some practical hints on the best means of ventilating barracks and other public buildings in India. I have taken here a wider view of the question of sanitation, and in the following pages have treated the subject under its several heads, in the order of their importance according to what appear to be, under existing circumstances, the requirements of the British soldier in India; namely, fresh air and free ventilation, pure water and food, and improved conservancy.

Should any quotation be found in the following pages to which the author's name has not been duly appended, I hope he will consider the omission unintentional, for I have not all the books by me which I have read on the subject under consideration; but, to make amends for any omissions of this kind, I append at the end of this volume a list of some of the works I have read on the subject, and most cordially acknowledge my obligations to the authors for the information gleaned from their writings. To these works I would refer my readers for more minute details of the various subjects which I am attempting to discuss, than could be included in a short practical treatise of this kind.

London, September, 1864.

CONTENTS.

CHAPTER I.

AIR AND VENTILATION.

CHAPTER II.

VENTILATION OF BARRACKS AND TENTS.

CHAPTER III.

WATER.

CHAPTER IV.

FOOD.

CHAPTER V.

CONSERVANCY.

CHAPTER VI.

DRAINAGE.

CHAPTER VII.

SUPERVISION.

CHAPTER VIII.

CONSTRUCTION OF BARRACKS.

CHAPTER IX.

FINANCIAL RESULTS.

CHAPTER X.

DESCRIPTION OF VARIOUS APPARATUS.

CHAPTER XI.

PRISONS AND PRISON-DISCIPLINE.

ERRATA.

Page 24, line 11, *for* "foul air of the barracks," *read* "foul air of the barrack."
,, 41, line 15, *for* "three-inch tatties," *read* "three such tatties."
,, 41, foot-note, line 2 from bottom, *for* "from 150° to 120°," *read* "from 100° to 120°."
,, 54, line 9, *for* "tent and loops," *read* "tent by loops."
,, 57, line 2, *for* "Three fans," *read* "These fans."
,, 57, line 8, *for* "wall," *read* "walls."
,, 68, line 6 of description of Fig. 17, *for* "filtered reservoir," *read* "filter and reservoir."
,, 111, line 2 of description of Fig. 23, *for* "wall of urinal," *read* "divisional wall of urinal."
,, 112, line 6, *for* "quantity," *read* "quality."
,, 132, lines 10 and 11, *for* "eight lacs of rupees (8,60,000)," *read* "nine lacs of rupees (9,60,000)."
,, 142, lines 2 and 3, *for* "Superintendent-Surgeon," *read* "Superintending Surgeon."
,, 149, line 5 from bottom, *for* "by prepared," *read* "be prepared."

HYGIENE OF THE ARMY IN INDIA.

CHAPTER I.

AIR AND VENTILATION.

It may perhaps be difficult to determine, to the satisfaction of every one, which of the two—foul air or impure water—is, *per se*, most injurious in a sanitary point of view. One thing, however, is certain, that water absorbs not only atmospheric air abundantly, but also the gases, vapours, and organic matter which may be floating in it. Hence, wherever foul air exists, the water and food-substances exposed to it must partake of its impurities; and every individual who lives in an impure atmosphere, whether rendered so by exhalations from the human body, or by other gases and vapours, imbibes poisons of a most deleterious kind with every breath inhaled, and with every morsel of food and drop of water received into the stomach. An abundant supply of pure air is therefore of the greatest importance to the human economy.

Chemistry of the Atmosphere.

The atmosphere is usually described as a gaseous fluid, containing oxygen and nitrogen in the proportions of 21 of the former to 79 of the latter, with a trace of carbonic acid in every 100 parts by volume. It may, however, be convenient to give a more minute detail of its composition; and the following, by Dr. W. A. Miller, may be accepted as a fair average analysis of atmospheric air:—

"The atmosphere is a mechanical mixture of several gases, amongst which oxygen and nitrogen constitute the principal portions, and which, notwithstanding their difference in density, are, owing to the principle of diffusion, uniformly mixed with each other.

"In addition to oxygen and nitrogen, the atmosphere contains a certain proportion of carbonic acid, a variable but minute trace of ammonia, traces of nitric acid, of some compound of carbon and hydrogen, and frequently, in towns, a perceptible amount of sulphurous acid or of sulphuretted hydrogen. Aqueous vapour is, of course, also present at all times, although its amount is liable to extensive fluctuations.

"The proportion of carbonic acid in the atmosphere varies from 3 to 6 parts in 10,000 of air. Saussure found that within these limits its amount is lessened after rain, owing to the solvent action of the descending shower, which carries a portion of the gas with it to the earth. During the night it increases, and diminishes again after sunrise. It is more abundant in densely-populated districts than in the open country. In inhabited dwellings, and in rooms for public assemblies, the proportion of carbonic acid may, however, greatly exceed the normal amount.

"The quantity of ammonia and nitric acid is

materially diminished after long-continued and heavy rains. Occasionally, from local and accidental circumstances, other gases and vapours are also met with. The air of towns contains, in addition, certain organic impurities in suspension.

"The average composition of the atmosphere may be stated as follows, in 100 parts by volume: —Oxygen, 20·61; nitrogen, 77·95; carbonic acid, ·04; aqueous vapour, 1·40; and traces of nitric acid, ammonia, carburetted hydrogen, sulphuretted hydrogen, and sulphurous acid."*

On account of the extreme heat, heavy periodical rains, frequent and heavy electrical discharges, and other local causes, the atmosphere of India is very liable to sudden changes, and most probably to variations in the relative volumes of some of its component gases; but the above analysis will be sufficient for our present purpose, and will show how readily mephitic gases, vapours, and organic impurities may be mixed up and suspended in the atmosphere.

Atmospheric Impurities: Animal Exhalations, and their Effects on Health.

With regard to impurities in the atmosphere, our information is, unfortunately, very limited; and beyond the fact that impure air contains a large increase in volume of carbonic acid, with, under certain conditions, a proportionate decrease of oxygen, traces of carburetted hydrogen, sulphuretted hydrogen, sulphurous acid, phosphoretted hydrogen,

---

* Miller's "Elements of Chemistry," Vol. II.

and carbonic oxyde, very little is known of their nature. In so far as the above gases are concerned, however, the air of crowded apartments, rendered impure by exhalations from the human body, partakes very much of the character of what is usually called malaria (or, more strictly speaking, miasm, according to Liebig's definition of the term), in its more confined acceptation, whether it arise from emanations from marshes or from other affected places. As in the case of miasm, great diversity of opinion exists regarding the true character of the exhalations of the living human body; but the chief part of the arguments are in favour of the vitiating principle, consisting of decomposing organic matters or gases, evolved by them.*

Whatever may be the analytical composition of foul air, rendered so by exhalations from the human body, we know that it contains a very large amount of organic matters. Dr. R. Angus Smith estimates

---

* Dr. T. H. Barker states in the Fothergillian Prize Essay for 1859, on the authority of Dr. Mason Good, "that the decomposition of the effluvium transmitted from the living body produces a miasm similar to that generated by the decomposition of dead organised matter, and hence capable of becoming a cause of fever under the influence of like agents. Fever thus excited is varied or modified by many of the same incidents that modify the miasmatic principle when issuing from dead organised matters; and hence a like diversity of type and vehemence. The miasm of human effluvium is chiefly distinguishable from that of dead organised matters by being less volatile, and having a power of more directly exhausting or debilitating the sensorial energy, when once received into the system; whence the fevers generated in gaols or other confined or crowded places contaminate the atmosphere to a less distance than the emanations from marshes and other swamps, but act with a greater degree of depression on the living fibre. The more stagnant the atmosphere, the more accumulated the miasmatic corpuscles, from whatever source derived; and the more accumulated the corpuscles, the more general the disease."

the amount of "animal matter, in the form of a putrescible albuminoid substance, at three parts in every 1000 by volume of respired air alone;" but the actual amount of organic matter given off by the whole of the human body in a given time has not been determined with a sufficient degree of accuracy to form a standard. Including, however, that given off by the skin, and judging from the quantity of perspiration exhaled in twenty-four hours in temperate climates, estimated by Lavoisier and Seguin at thirty-three ounces in twenty-four hours,* the amount of organic matter given off by the combined action of the lungs and skin in a hot climate like that of India must be very great indeed.

It is universally admitted that the exhalations from the human body are of a highly putrescible nature;†

---

* "The repetition of Lavoisier and Seguin's experiments during a long period showed that, during a state of rest, the average loss by cutaneous and pulmonary exhalation, in a minute, is from seventeen to eighteen grains; and that, of the eighteen grains, eleven pass off by the skin and seven by the lungs."—(Kirkes's "Hand-book of Physiology.") "The solid non-volatile constituents of the sweat have been found to range between about 0·5 and 1·25 per cent. . . . Among the solid constituents, chloride of sodium is the most abundant. Lactates, butyrates, and acetates of ammonia and soda are also present, besides small quantities of phosphate of lime. . . . Carbonic acid and nitrogen are likewise exhaled from the surface of the body in considerable quantity, particularly the former. The sweat contains also a quantity of a peculiar azotised matter, very prone to decomposition, as well as an odorous principle. The cutaneous excretion from the general surface of the body has almost invariably an acid reaction, owing to the presence of free lactic acid; but the excretion from the axillæ and the feet is sometimes found to be alkaline."—(Miller's "Elements of Chemistry," vol. iii.) Urea is said to be one of the ordinary constituents of the fluid of perspiration. According to some authorities, the acidity of perspiration depends chiefly on formic acid.

† "When the vapour contained in the air of crowded and over-heated rooms is artificially condensed by means of cold surfaces, and collected, it is

and doubtless the extreme rapidity with which they pass into this condition, is owing to the finely-divided state in which the organic matters come into contact with the oxygen of the air, in consequence of which they become oxidised immediately on their separation from the living body. And who can fully estimate the baneful effects of the introduction into the system of putrid animal matters? We see that wounds, be they ever so slight, received in dissecting the dead human body, produce most serious consequences through the introduction into the system of a very minute quantity of some very virulent poison, generated during the first stage of decomposition; and, supposing that the organic matter given off by the living body partakes of the nature of this poison, immediately when decomposition begins, (and there is nothing impossible in this, seeing that in both cases we have to deal with human organic matters in the first stage of putrefaction), we shall only be surprised

---

found to be highly impregnated with matter of an albuminous nature, which is extremely likely to become putrid. Moisture so obtained, on being evaporated, gives out a strong smell of perspiration; and the dry residue, when exposed to heat, emits an odour of burning flesh."—(H. B. Condy, on "Air and Water and their Impurities.") At page 21 of Dr. Barker's essay, already quoted, it is stated:—"Liebig further remarks:—'All the observations hitherto made upon gaseous contagious matters prove that they also are substances in a state of decomposition. When vessels filled with ice are placed in air impregnated with gaseous contagious matter, their outer surfaces become covered with water containing a certain amount of this matter in solution. This water soon becomes putrid, and, in common language, putrefies; or, to describe the change more correctly, the process of decomposition of the dissolved contagious matter is completed in the water.' All gases emitted from putrefying animal and vegetable substances in process of disease generally possess a peculiar nauseous offensive smell; a circumstance which in most cases proves the presence of a body in a state of decomposition, that is, of chemical action."

that the mischief arising from such a poison being brought into contact with the blood, as it circulates through the lungs, has not a more rapidly fatal result.

This is an extreme view of the case; but we know that, when ordinary putrid matter is brought into contact with other substances, not at the time, nor, perhaps, at all in themselves putrescible, they rapidly become so; and this is particularly the case if they contain any of the constituents of the decomposing substance.* We have no reason to suppose that any substance given off from the blood in its passage through the lungs could not be received back into the blood through the same channel, provided it be presented in an equally finely-divided or gaseous state. Now, this is exactly what takes place with the foul air of over-crowded and ill-ventilated apartments; and, assuming this to be correct (and I think there can be no doubt of it), the danger attending the re-introduction into the blood of one of its own constituents in a putrid state must be very great, as tending to set up the putrefactive process in the whole mass of the circulating fluid. In what other way does the foul air of over-crowded apartments produce the low type of typhoid fever usually known as gaol fever? And what other diseases may not be induced by a poison which has proved fatal, in many lamentable instances, in a few hours?

In addition to the noxious gases and other matters already noticed, it may not be too much to assume

---

* Liebig's "Chemistry of Agriculture."

that a portion of the gases which constitute atmospheric air may, on coming into contact with the exhalations from the body, form other substances not at present recognised, but, at the same time, highly noxious in a sanitary point of view. However, it is unnecessary for our present purpose to speculate further on the probable substances supposed to constitute the active principle of impure air poison. That foul air does exist in close and crowded apartments, as well as in the open air in low confined localities, and becomes a slow or a rapid poison, according to circumstances, we have too sure proof; and as surely as the human constitution is subjected to its baneful influence, so surely must debility, impaired health, and eventually death, in some shape, ensue. The only way of preventing every person from being the means of poisoning himself, is to keep the body constantly surrounded with pure air; for, however faultless all other sanitary arrangements may be, without a sufficient supply of pure air he must, within a certain period, be poisoned by the exhalations from his own body, and die in consequence, as surely as if he had taken an overdose of any other poison.

The organs of smell point out that foul air, even under favourable circumstances, does not readily leave the vicinity of the body, but, on the contrary, continues floating within a few feet of the place where it is generated; and, unless it be freely diluted with fresh atmospheric air, or carried off altogether, the body soon becomes enveloped in an atmosphere rendered poisonous by its own exhalations.

Diurnal Atmospheric Movements in India: their Effect in Disease.

In India the atmosphere is subject to certain daily periodical variations or movements, which occur with considerable regularity, and of which the following is a brief account.

During the dry hot months and intervals of dry weather in the rainy season of the upper provinces of India, which comprise at least seven months of the year, after a period of eight or nine hours of dead calm, commencing about 6 or 7 o'clock p.m. and continuing to about 3 or 4 a.m., the atmosphere begins to show signs of motion, in light puffs from the W. and N.W.; and by 5 or half-past 5 a.m. these puffs have become a steady light breeze from the W.N.W. This gradually increases in force till after the sun has some time passed the meridian, and generally gains its maximum strength about 2 p.m., after which it gradually decreases till 6 or 7 o'clock p.m. A dead calm then again succeeds; and one feels that, in addition to coolies to pull the punkah, a greater luxury still would be two or three to do the work of breathing. During this calm period natural ventilation will not proceed, let the means be what they may; and it is during this period that foul-air poisoning proceeds silently and surely.

But the quantity of poison actually received into the system through the lungs and other channels is not the only bad result arising from deficient ventilation during the hours in question. Between 2 and 3 o'clock a.m. a sudden change takes place in the atmosphere, more or less perceptible to the outward senses; and although it is not always indicated by the thermometer, the sensation is one of a decided fall in temperature of the air. Persons who have passed a restless night on account of excessive heat, will generally fall asleep under this agreeable change; and, as the air begins to move about the same time, individuals so situated, if sleeping outside or with open doors, are very soon under the full influence of a draught. What, then, must be the consequence with those who have been bathed in perspiration for six or seven hours, and whose vital action has been reduced to a very low ebb by the inhalation of foul air saturated with poisonous matter? Such is the condition of the inmates of our European barracks in Upper India. The doors and windows of these barracks are always open, and whatever changes take place in the movement and temperature of the air outside must, to a certain extent, be communicated to that inside, and the inmates, who have passed a restless, sleepless night, enveloped in foul air, deriving temporary relief from the change in question, fall asleep almost always in a draught of more or less strength; at all events, in a considerably cooler atmosphere than they had been experiencing for hours before. The consequences of this must be sudden chills and checked perspiration, resulting in serious constitutional disturbance.

The cause of the change alluded to, which, though not so marked, occurs also at the same hour in the afternoon, has not been fully determined, but it is about the time indicated that atmospheric pressure and electric tension are at their minimum; and it would appear that the vital action is also at its minimum about the same time. At least, this much we know, that it is about this time that the depression, and not unfrequently fatal collapse, takes place after exacerbations of fever. So satisfied am I on this point, from long experience, that, whenever I have had a severe case of fever to deal with, let the type be what it may, I have invariably given orders to be called at 2 o'clock a.m., and never considered it safe to leave my patient until an hour after the depression had passed off. The depression is not confined to the fevers of tropical climates. I have often seen the same result in typhus and other fevers in Europe.*

According to my experience, it is about the time in question that the incubation of cholera and other epidemic diseases takes place. I have almost invariably found that persons suffering from cholera, state, if carefully questioned, that they felt restless some time during the night, and had a copious evacuation; after which they felt better, and slept quietly till about six o'clock, when they were suddenly seized with uneasiness, and an earnest desire to go again to stool. On more closely questioning, I have found that the first disturbance occurred about, or a little before, three o'clock. I have often seen the second disturbance, or what is more generally called the first symptoms of cholera, postponed till seven or eight o'clock, and even later, when the disease was not of a very virulent type.

* Children suffering from fever should be most carefully watched at the time alluded to, and a stimulant should be at hand to give at once if necessary, as in their case, particularly if the collapse fairly set in, restoration will be very difficult.

I feel convinced that, during the prevalence of epidemic cholera, the symptoms described above are indicative of very serious mischief; and I consider that every person seized with such symptoms about the time indicated should be carefully watched during the whole of the following day, if not actually put under treatment. In this stage, cholera is as amenable to treatment as any other disease. If a mild opiate, with a little calomel or blue pill, were administered, with a cup of warm tea or a small dose of diffusible stimulant, such as a few grains of sesquicarbonate of ammonia, in any convenient vehicle, or a little weak warm brandy and water, at the time of the first disturbance, a great portion of the cases which subsequently prove of a serious nature would never assume any severe form.

Impure Air and Water as Exciting Causes of Epidemic Disease.

Impure air and water may not be the only causes of cholera, dysentery, diarrhœa, and epidemic fevers; but when the source of these impurities is the exhalations from the human body, they are most powerful exciting causes of these diseases. The benefit which is derived from removal into camp or change of quarters during visitations of cholera and other epidemics, arises chiefly from two causes; first, the cutting off of the supply of poison; and secondly, the dilution of the poison already in the system, by an unlimited supply of pure air and water. The duration of the epidemic will depend on the extent of poisoning which has taken place previously to removal; on the space, or, in other words, the quantity of pure air allotted night and day to the affected in their new quarters; and on the power remaining of eliminating the poison already imbibed.

Cholera and other epidemic diseases generally appear in certain groups of men at almost fixed periods; sometimes at one season, sometimes at another; but almost always after the affected have been unduly exposed to foul air from bad ventilation, over-crowding in their dwelling places, or the massing together of large numbers of human beings, which, even in the open air, will contaminate the atmosphere for some distance, as at large fairs* and in large standing camps, where great numbers of people are congregated.

During the cold season, when soldiers are either on parade, or otherwise employed on duty or amusement in the open air almost the whole day, the foul air poison taken into the system during the previous hot season is thrown off to a certain extent, and they are, comparatively speaking, healthy, and continue so until again confined to the precincts of their ill-ventilated barracks; when cholera, dysentery, diarrhœa, or fever towards the middle and end of the hot weather, are almost the invariable consequence.

---

* After the Hurdwar and other large fairs in India, cholera almost always appears in the villages on the lines of roads leading from them; but the cases are generally confined to people who have been at these fairs. For instance, at Deyrah Dhoon, about 40 miles from Hurdwar, there are often two annual visitations of cholera; viz., one in April or May, confined to individuals returning from the Hurdwar fair; and one later in the season, of the usual epidemic type, among the general inhabitants of the town.

The same arguments hold good with regard to all the other groups of human beings in India. The lazy villager, if not employed in his fields, will seek the sunny side of his hut to bask in the warmth of the sun's rays; and even the prisoner, immured within the walls of his prison, is more out of doors, and breathes much more fresh air, during the cold season than in the hot and rainy months of the year; and, in consequence, like the others, enjoys much better health, until again more closely confined to his barracks, when, if not allowed sufficient space, he suffers from all the evils arising from foul-air poison.

However various and severe may be the peculiarities attending visitations of epidemic cholera at different times and seasons, there is one circumstance which is never wanting, namely, the severity of the disease in point of numbers attacked, and virulence of type among those who have been living in the most crowded and ill-ventilated dwellings. Numerous instances of this fact could be cited, but I will confine myself to two: During the awful visitation of cholera at Lahore, in 1861, while the men of the Foot Regiments were dying in hundreds, those of the Artillery, quartered in the Fort, had a remarkable immunity from the disease. The medical officer in charge accounted for this by the men being less crowded. He states:—"They were less crowded in the barracks, and the building occupied by them is, upon the whole, the best in the Fort." Again, on the same occasion, two officers of the 51st Foot were attacked with cholera in the Fort; and it is stated that their quarters were "small and the ventilation insufficient."*

The baneful influence of impure air on the human constitution is so well understood generally, that some may think it superfluous to discuss this part of the subject at such length; but has everyone whose duty it is to see that, in addition to other points of sanitation, those intrusted to his care are not poisoned by the exhalations from their own bodies, fully considered the subject, and arrived at the important fact that, however complete other sanitary arrangements may be, if the subtle poison of foul air be present, it will frustrate his best endeavours in the prevention of disease, and in curing it if once established.

It is very common in the present day to regard impure water as the chief source of epidemic disease. No one will dispute for a moment the great danger to health arising from the use of impure water; but what I would contend for is that, before attributing any disease or group of diseases to this cause alone, the true source of the impurities should be carefully ascertained. Let us admit, by way of illustration, that during the prevalence of an epidemic a large amount of organic matter is found in the water used by the affected, and that the air breathed by them also contains the same impurities, would a supply of pure water remove or avert the evil while the foul air remained? Certainly not.† The composition of air

* Report of the Commissioners appointed to inquire into the Cholera Epidemic of 1861.

† Fortunately we are in possession of a substance (thanks to Mr. Condy and Dr. Angus Smith for its introduction) as an air-test, by which impurities

and water is, in no small degree, the same, and they become poisoned very much in the same way; but "the blood will become much more readily poisoned through the lungs than through the stomach."*

Cholera in Indian Prisons: Results of Over-crowding.

With regard to the true cause of epidemic cholera, unfortunately very little is known; but the theory that it is something which has a very depressing effect on the nervous system generally, is supported by a greater amount of evidence than any of the other theories. And what can have a more depressing effect than inhalation of foul air? In accordance with this view, I shall give a few facts, which, to my mind, point to foul-air poison as one of the direct causes of epidemic disease, which, under certain conditions, not at present recognised, assumes the choleraic type; and then proceed to explain what I consider the best means of getting rid of foul air as it exists in the quarters of the British soldier in India.

Prior to the concentration of prisoners in large prisons in the North-West Provinces, each district jail had its full complement of inmates; and cholera, dysentery, and diarrhœa, were in a measure endemic in these jails; but since all the long-term prisoners, that is, about two-thirds of the total number, have

---

in the atmosphere can be detected as readily as impurities in water. An apparatus for the purpose will be described hereafter.

* Dr. Angus Smith's Evidence before the Indian Sanitary Commission.

been removed to central prisons, these diseases rarely appear in district jails in an epidemic form. I was upwards of nine years in medical charge of district jails, and never saw but one case of cholera among the prisoners; while at the same time visitations of the disease were just as rife and severe among the free population in the neighbourhood as at other stations. Again, at the central prisons, where the prisoners are massed together in great numbers, visitations of cholera and other epidemic diseases are frequent and severe, particularly whenever the prisons become in the least degree crowded. The conservancy and general management of these prisons are quite as carefully attended to as at the district jails, perhaps more so; but in the latter case the prisoners, being few, and confined in barracks constructed originally for three times their number, live, comparatively speaking, in a pure atmosphere.

The regulation space allowed in the prisons of the North-Western Provinces, is 500 cubic feet to each prisoner; and a reference to the Prison Returns will show that hitherto, whenever the number in confinement has amounted to anything over the full complement, an epidemic of some kind—generally cholera—has always made its appearance, and carried off large numbers of the prisoners. Again, whenever the number has been considerably under the regulation complement, the inmates have been free from cholera, and exempt generally from other epidemic diseases. I think that data might be found, in the returns of these prisons, to show that the germs of cholera do not lie in store from previous visitations, ready to spring up, like mushrooms in a bed, at a moment's notice, without any known cause; and that the disease is not communicated by the direct application of the excrementitious matter of the affected so constantly as some authorities would wish us to believe. It would be found that cases of cholera occur among the prisoners as amongst other groups of individuals; but that the disease never assumes a severe type except during or after over-crowding; and, further, that outbreaks of the disease among the prisoners do not necessarily follow previous visitations, even during severe epidemics among the troops and free population at the same stations, so long as the prisons have not been over-crowded for some time previously to the appearance of the disease among the population outside their walls.

An instance occurred lately in this country, which will prove instructive in regard to the question under consideration: "At Festiniog, in Merionethshire, a village favourably situated on the side of the adjacent mountain range, where the air is pure, the rainfall easily carried off, and the inhabitants hitherto usually healthy, a fever broke out, and prevailed to such an extent as to demand inquiry by the Government authorities. It was found, that within the last two years the great demand for labour at the slate-quarries in the neighbourhood had brought an accession of population to the place, far exceeding the accommodation available in the way of lodgings; and over-crowding in the cottages, to a most pernicious extent, was the consequence. In cottages containing two low rooms, eight feet by six and twelve feet by six respectively, ten, and even twelve, people were found to be lodged. The work in the quarries was continued day and night, by relays of labourers, and in like manner were the lodgings occupied; the bed which one left to go to his labour being immediately tenanted by another whose labour was done. It is unnecessary to speculate on the origin or cause of the fever; if Festiniog had been inhabited by none but its original population, no epidemic would have been heard of in the place."

If we turn to the Report of the Army Medical Department for 1861, we shall find many well-authenticated instances, particularly among the troops serving in the Mediterranean, of the increase of zymotic diseases resulting from overcrowding and defective ventilation. No one, of course, will dispute the evils likely to arise from bad drainage and other kinds of defective conservancy; but when the barrack accommodation is under 400 cubic feet per man, or even when, with nearly double this amount, large numbers are congregated together in the same apartment, in a hot climate particularly, the best conservancy will not prevent the inevitable consequences of overcrowding and imperfect supply of air.

Imperfect Ventilation of Tents.

However poisonous the atmosphere of barracks may be, it is mild in comparison with that of tents. The space contained in each of the largest tents usually supplied for the use of European soldiers does not exceed 2,850 cubic feet; and as one tent is allowed to every twenty-five men, the space per head is 114 cubic feet; but, allowing for absentees on sentry and fatigue duties, &c., the space per man will not exceed at most 125 cubic feet, a quantity of air totally inadequate for the support of human life in a healthy condition. Hence, during long marches, particularly at seasons when the men cannot remain outside their tents, the system becomes more completely saturated with foul air poison, than when they live stationary in even the worst constructed barracks; and to this may be attributed, in a great measure, the severe visitations of cholera and other epidemics, which occur so frequently after long marches, even although these be undertaken and continued, to all appearance, under favourable circumstances.

Because the temperature in tents is high during the day time and low at night, it does not follow that this arises from the free access of the external air to the interior of them. The canvas walls of a tent are almost as impervious to air as the brick walls of a barrack, and absorb moisture much more readily; and, if it be borne in mind that expired air, when it leaves the lungs, is almost completely saturated with moisture, carrying with it a large quantity of organic matter which passes quickly into a putrid state, it will be seen that the cloth of a tent must very soon become charged with foul air poison, and consequently a ready source of great mischief. The few openings close to the ground and about the eaves, which, by the by, are generally carefully closed, go a very little way in relieving the effects of the excessive over-crowding, so that the free ventilation of tents is as essentially necessary as, or indeed more so than, that of barracks, while the space per man is confined to 125 cubic feet. Who, that has experienced it, will ever forget the fœtid odour that greets him on first entering a tent which has been crowded for six or seven hours with human beings? The nearest approach to it, is the effluvium of an ill-ventilated dissection-room.

There is another evil attending the life of the common soldier in tents; namely, he has no sleeping cot. His bed is simply made on the ground, with a little straw, or grass at most, spread under it, so that the foul air has no opportunity of escaping; and even the little fresh air that may gain ingress to the tent has not free access to him, and he lies the whole night completely enveloped in an atmosphere composed of the fœtid gases and vapours exhaled from his own body. Can it then be wondered at, that men who have passed so many hours in such a foul atmosphere feel seriously fatigued, after a short march of only ten or twelve miles, and remain listless and inactive during the rest of the day? Yet nothing of a practical nature in the ventilation of tents has yet been carried into effect.

In the next chapter, I shall describe the means of ventilating barracks and tents.

CHAPTER II.

VENTILATION OF BARRACKS AND TENTS.

It is stated "that probably between four and five hundred cubic feet of air pass through the lungs daily;" and "the size of an apartment, therefore, in which persons are confined, should be such, and its ventilation should be so arranged, that each individual may be supplied with the above quantity of pure air as a minimum."* Now, under certain conditions of the atmosphere, this can only be effected by setting the air in motion by artificial means. If the atmosphere be perfectly still, and the temperature outside and inside a building containing a number of men be the same, or nearly so, no current can be established naturally in any direction, whatever the arrangements of the openings for the ingress and egress of air may be; and the inmates so situated are almost in a similar condition to that in which they would be, were each individual shut up in a small apartment containing much less cubic space than that which is allotted to him in the building.

Such is the condition of the inmates of our barracks in India during the calm, sultry nights of the hot and rainy seasons. I have on several occasions conducted experiments in barracks well

---

* Todd and Bowman's "Physiology," Vol. II., page 410.

provided with openings for the ingress and egress of air, with the view of testing the state of ventilation; and, with the lightest substances I could procure, the external atmosphere being calm and above 80°, have failed in discovering any movement in the air inside.* Indeed, during this state of the atmosphere, even smoke ascends very slowly in the open air; and the breathing is oppressed, and performed with more or less difficulty.

Ventilation is much more difficult, even in temperate climates, during summer than in winter, on account of the difference of temperature between the internal and external air being much less than in cold weather. How, then, can it be expected that natural ventilation will proceed in the climate of India, when both temperatures are the same, or nearly so, and not unfrequently the internal the lowest? Even if we admit, for argument's sake, that the external air is cooler than the internal, still a few degrees in difference of temperature will not establish a sufficiently strong current to carry off the noxious exhalations from the human body; some of them may, perhaps, ascend a certain distance, but, the current being feeble, the foul air is cooled before its exit from the building, and descends, to be again inspired. Punkahs will, to a certain extent, set the air in motion, and thereby

* A very convenient mode of ascertaining the direction of currents of air, is by setting fire to a small piece of thick brown paper, which has been dried after having been saturated with a solution of nitrate of potass. The paper gives out a quantity of beautiful blue smoke, which will of course take the direction of any movement in the air; and, as it burns slowly, the observation may be continued by the same person for any length of time, and at several points of an apartment within a very short period.

cool the body through increasing the evaporation of the moisture on its surface; but they do not expel the air from the interior of buildings, nor reduce its temperature in the least degree; and in the case of apartments filled with human beings, allowing about sixty square feet to each individual (which is above the average area per head in most of the old barracks in the North-West Provinces), they simply mix up the air of the apartment; so that, instead of each person breathing the exhalations of his own body, he inhales the general foul air of the barracks.

The new barracks recently erected have an ample number of openings for the ingress and egress of air, such as doors, windows, open ridges, &c.; still, when they are occupied by the regulation number of men, the air during the night-time is foul and poisonous. It is generally supposed that the air in those barracks is always pure and sweet; but such opinion can only have been gathered from day inspections in the cool weather, when the barracks have been empty during two or three hours. I consider that no barrack, containing the regulation number of inmates, and not possessing other means of ventilation than the usual openings for the ingress and egress of air, is ever, during the hot sultry months of the year, or, perhaps, at any time, free from a poisonous quantity of foul air at night.*

* I have, with the view of gaining information on points of improvement, or of mistakes to be avoided in ventilation and sanitation generally, visited a great portion of the barracks in the North-West Provinces, and feel confident that very few of them are ever entirely free of foul air, even in the daytime. What, then, must be the state of the air during the calm still hours of night, when every available place is occupied, and not a breath of air stirring?

Those residents in India who have no better means of procuring fresh air than those afforded by natural channels, pass restless nights, enveloped in foul air and bathed in perspiration, the arrest of which, by the atmospheric changes taking place in the early morning, results in seriously impaired health, and not unfrequently in acute disease, ultimately terminating in death. "It is," says Sir J. R. Martin, "during sleep that alternations of heat and cold most seriously affect us;" arising, no doubt, from the action of atmospheric changes on the surface of the body, at the time when the vital power is at its minimum tension, and when, consequently, the equilibrium of the sympathies which exist between the skin and internal organs is more easily deranged.* To provide against these sudden

* "The regulation of the temperature of the body is only one of the purposes fulfilled by perspiration; another important one is the removal from the system of a number of compounds noxious to animal life. It was estimated by Lavoisier and Séguin that eleven grains of perspiration were exhaled from the skin in the course of a minute, a quantity which is equivalent to thirty-three ounces in twenty-four hours." Mr. Erasmus Wilson estimates the length of the tube of the perspiratory system of the whole surface of the body at 48,600 yards, or nearly 28 miles. Well may the talented author exclaim, What if this drainage were obstructed? Krause estimates the total number of perspiratory glands at 2,381,248; and, supposing the orifice of each gland to present a surface of 1-500th of an inch diameter, he reckons that the whole of the glands would present an evaporating surface of about eight square inches. The watery exhalation from the glands, however, probably forms but a very small part of the total amount. Milne-Edwards estimates it at not above one-sixth. The greater quantity must be furnished by simple transudation through the cuticle. The glands, however, doubtless eliminate the solid matters of the perspiration. These observations again bring us to the practical conclusion of Moseley, that cold is the cause of almost all the diseases of hot climates, to which climate alone is accessory. "Even in Europe the summer night affects us with a chill, while the same temperature a few months later in the winter season would feel oppressive from its heat."—Martin on the "Influence of Tropical Climates," pp. 89 and 90.

changes and chills, it is simply necessary to establish about the body a regular circulation of pure atmospheric air, at an even and moderate temperature; and at the same time to cut off all sources of unequal currents and draughts by closed doors and windows. In a cold climate, the air must be tempered by artificial heat. There will then be no sudden chills; for this reason, that the body will have been kept at an even temperature, and the amount of evaporation from its surface uniform throughout the night, by the air circulating round it having been of a steady pressure and temperature. There will be the usual fall in temperature in the early morning, it is true; but the effect will be no more than—in fact, for reasons already mentioned, not so much as—that experienced in the well-ventilated rooms of the better classes.

It is a well-known fact, that the most healthy men in India are those who provide themselves with large, well-ventilated bedrooms, and sleep invariably with closed doors and windows. The habits of most of the different groups of Europeans in India are not so widely different, with this one exception, as to account for the frightful sickness and mortality confined to one of these groups. Some of them eat the same kind of food, drink the same kind of water, and are, in some instances, not less intemperate; yet they do not suffer in the same degree; but then they have an abundance of fresh air. It then becomes absolutely incumbent on those who have the charge of the suffering group, to remedy so palpable an evil without delay.

If we turn to the medical statistics of the British Army serving in India, furnished by the several authorities on this important subject, we find that the average percentage of deaths to strength from cholera, in European regiments in the Bengal Presidency, for the eight years ending 1853-54, was 0·1 among officers to 7·0 among men.* This of itself shows that there is some preventable influence among the men, other than merely the water which they use; for in most cases the water used by both officers and men, if not procured from the same surface-source, is obtained from wells not very far apart.

But, to return to the question of a sufficient supply of fresh air, a steady circulation of pure air can be maintained day and night by the machinery and apparatus to be described, in a given number of barracks, from one end of the year to the other. And, as it has been shown that the supply will be ample for all purposes, every barrack should be fitted with proper doors and glass windows, so as to provide for the sufficient lighting of the interior of the buildings—a most essential sanitary need, very much neglected in our Indian barracks. The inmates would thus be enabled to live day and night in a pure atmosphere, of even temperature, equal, and in fact superior, to what is enjoyed by their, at present, more fortunate European brethren in the country. It is hardly necessary to add, that the mode of ventilation, which will be presently described, implies strict attention to closure of the doors and windows of the barracks at

* Dr. Hugh Macpherson's Analysis of later Medical Returns.

night and during the heat of the day; in fact, the barracks should be managed in every way in this respect as the private houses of the better classes.

As matters now stand in India, a few moments' reflection will convince the most casual observer that, independently of other advantages, the introduction of such a system of ventilation would prove of immense financial interest in rendering existing barracks, many of which must be condemned for no other reason than want of proper ventilation, not only habitable but healthy.

It may be admitted that, let the ventilation be what it may, large bodies of men should not be congregated in the same apartment day and night; and it would perhaps be right, that not more than twenty men should occupy the same apartment at one time. It is held that, to provide for the thorough ventilation of a barrack, or hut, for even this small number, the building must be detached. Now in the "plenum method," which I maintain, on the grounds already advanced, to be the only one that can provide for thorough ventilation in the climate of India, it is not necessary that small apartments should be detached buildings; so that, in existing barracks, divided by divisional cross-walls into rooms, each sufficient for twenty men or a smaller number, every apartment could be thoroughly ventilated by the plan in question, and, in point of fresh air, rendered as healthy as if it stood by itself in an open plain.

In the preceding remarks it has been demonstrated, firstly, that in hot climates natural ventilation will not proceed during certain atmospheric conditions;

and, secondly, that however well an apartment may be supplied with doors, windows, &c., no movement in the internal air takes place during these conditions, at least not sufficient to change the atmosphere completely. Ventilation by artificial means must be employed; otherwise the inmates must suffer. No plan hitherto in use can effect this most desirable end so well as propulsion of the air by properly arranged fans. It has been very properly urged that, "if fresh air will not go where we wish it we must drive it; and, instead of trusting to languid currents, created by indirect means for the ventilation of crowded apartments, it should be pumped in per force."

Apparatus for Ventilating Barracks.

Were the barracks in India built in several stories, and arranged in blocks sufficient for the accommodation of a whole regiment, on, comparatively speaking, a small area, ventilation on the plenum method would be a simple matter; but, as most of the existing buildings are only one story high, more or less distant from each other, and as in every instance the barracks for a whole regiment cover a considerable area, the economical ventilation of them becomes a more difficult affair.

Without actual experiment, it would be difficult to ascertain the exact quantity of air that could be forced through a system of ramifying flues, and discharged by a series of outlets into a number of apartments at uncertain distances from the propelling power. But, judging from what has already been done in this mode of ventilation, I have no doubt that two fans, driven by steam or bullock power,* which will discharge twenty thousand cubic feet of air per minute, with properly arranged flues, would be quite sufficient for the ventilation of barracks for a whole regiment, even as they exist at present in India; and, if specially constructed for this mode of ventilation, one fan would do the work.†

Supposing the barracks which are to be ventilated, arranged échelon, or otherwise extending a considerable distance in line, as barracks in India generally are (Fig. 1, N N, page 31), a system of underground masonry flues must be constructed, consisting of main flues (M M, Figs. 1 and 2 *a*), from which proceed, at proper intervals, barrack-flues (E E). The fans and other apparatus for supplying air at the end of the main flues should be placed to windward and about the middle of the line of buildings, 300 feet or more from the nearest barracks (Fig. 1). It is hardly necessary to mention that, were the fans placed nearer the buildings, the supply of pure air could not be ensured; in fact, foul air would often be returned by them. The main flues (M M) should have a transverse area of 4ft. 6in. by 3ft. The barrack-flues (E E) running under the floor in the middle of each building (Figs. 1 and 2), should not have a less diameter than

---

* This system of ventilation has been in operation, at the Agra Central Prison, for some time, and found to answer admirably. A common fan, worked by hand, the propeller of which is 3ft. 6in. in diameter, and its velocity under 300 revolutions per minute, is found quite sufficient for each corridor of 68 cells measuring 283 feet in length.

† There would be no difficulty in the application of bullock power; but, according to my experience, steam power would be more regular, and more economical in the end.

2ft. 6in. by 2ft. From each barrack-flue, within the building, proceeds a series of diffusion-pipes (F F, Figs. 1

FIG. 1.

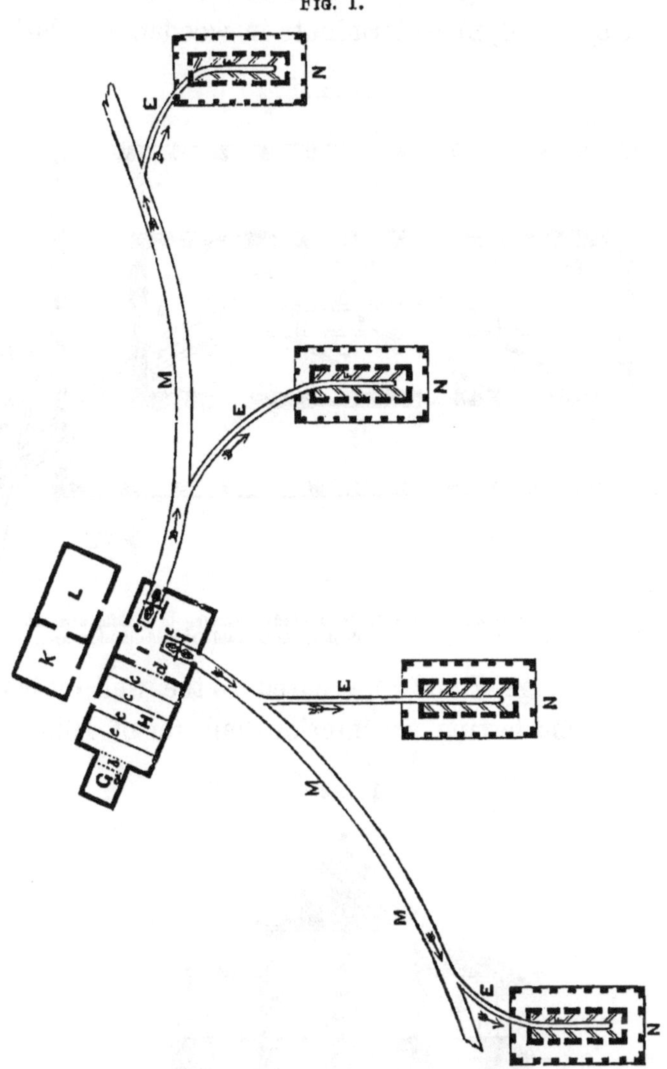

Fig. 1. Relative Position of Ventilating Apparatus to Flues, Barracks, &c. E E E, Barrack-flues. F F, Diffusion-pipes. G, Fresh air shaft. H, Cooling-room. I, Fan-room. K, Ice-making machine. L, Steam-engine. M M M, Main flues. N N N N, Barracks. *a*. Valve for admission of air to heating-room. *b*. Ditto to cooling-room. *c c c c* Khuss tatties. *e e* Fans.

and 2*a*), each nine inches in diameter, and made of earthenware. These pipes should be continued to the required height in the masonry of the walls (Fig. 2 *b*, C C, Fig. 4, B), or terminate in wooden ventilating

FIG. 2 *a*.

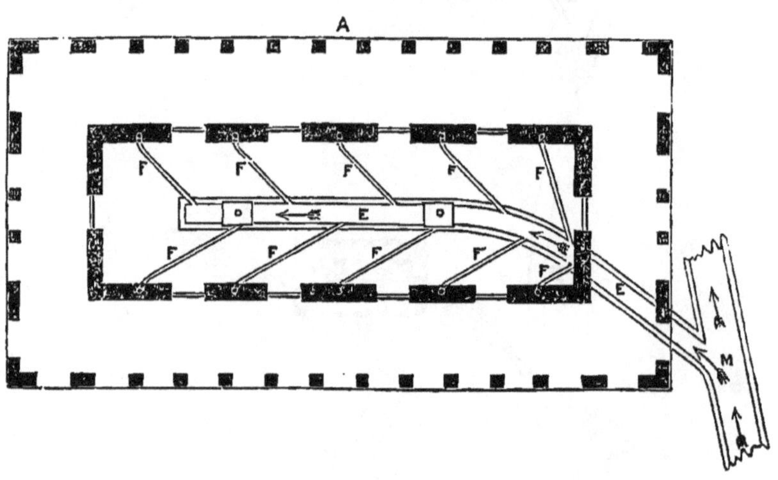

A. Ground Plan of accommodation for twenty beds according to existing barracks. E. Barrack-flue. F F, Diffusion-pipes. M. Main flue. O O, Table-shaped diffusion-cases.

cases (D, Figs. 7 and 8), secured to the wall by iron clamps, and having an interior diameter of 10in. by

FIG. 2 *b*.

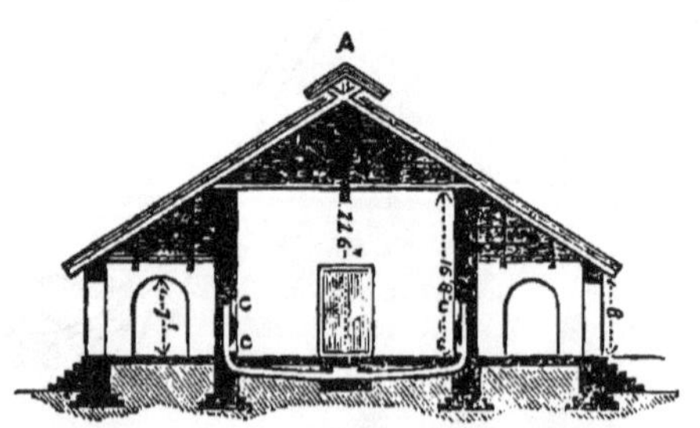

Sectional end view of ditto. A. Ridge-ventilator. C C. Diffusion-openings.

5in. The air escapes from the pipes in the wall, or from the ventilating cases, by means of a series of exit-openings (c c, Figs. 2*b*, 2*c*, 3, 4, 5, and 6). These openings must be covered with perforated zinc plates, of a watch-glass shape, or convex outwardly (Fig 4, c), so as to diffuse the air in much the same way as

Fig. 2 *c*.

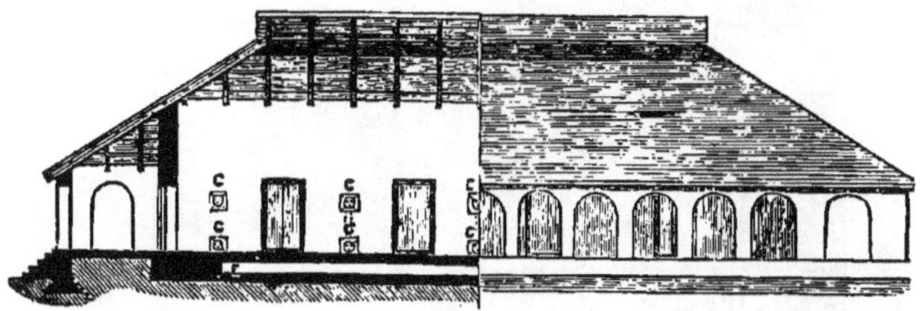

Elevation and partial longitudinal section of barrack. C. C. Diffusion-openings.

water is thrown from the rose on the spout of a watering-pot. These openings should be at the apex

Fig. 3.

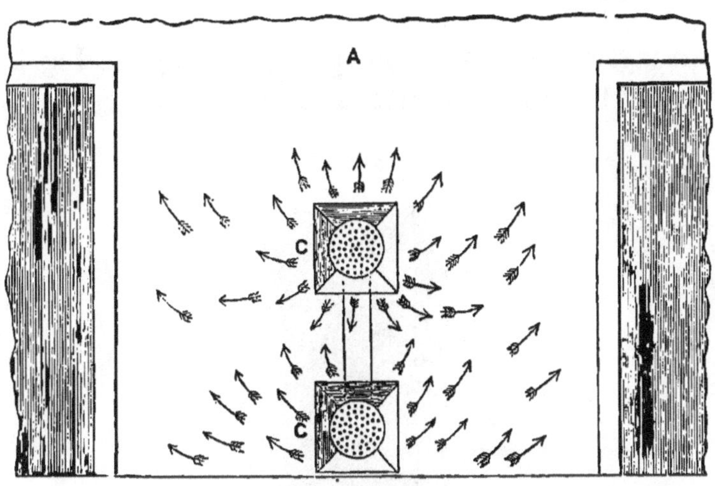

A. Elevation of portion of interior wall of a barrack. C. Exit opening for fresh air, covered with perforated metal. The arrows indicate the course of the air.

of funnel-shaped cavities in the wall, which gradually expand to a diameter of twelve inches at the mouth or base, and are there protected by iron grating (Fig.

5). A section of a portion of wall, giving the

Fig. 4. Fig. 5.

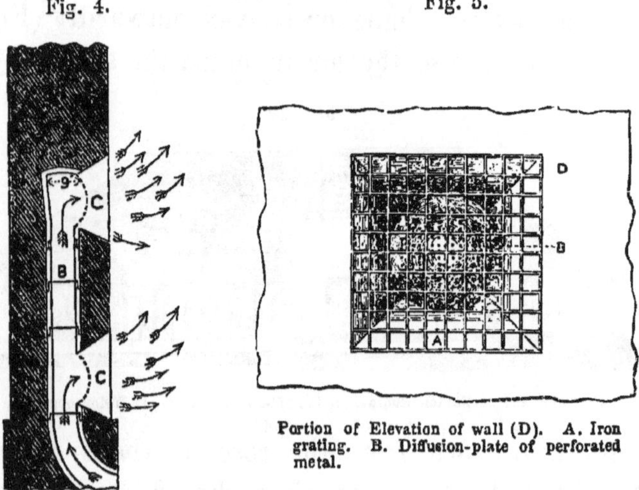

Portion of Elevation of wall (D). A. Iron grating. B. Diffusion-plate of perforated metal.

Section of Diffusion-pipe and opening. B. Diffusion-pipe. C. C. Diffusion openings. The arrows indicate the course of the current of air.

arrangement of a diffusion-opening, is shewn in Fig. 6. It will be seen from Figs. 2*a* and 2*c*, that the open-

Fig. 6.

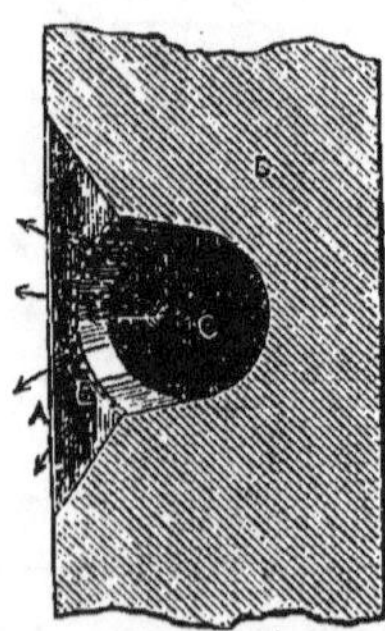

Section of portion of wall (D). A. Iron grating over diffusion-pipe. B. Perforated metal diffusion-plate. C. diffusion-pipe.

ings for the diffusion of air are arranged in the barracks in the space between the doors, and consequently between the men's sleeping-cots—one opening being close to the floor, and another four feet above it. The wooden ventilating cases, represented at D, Figs. 7 and 8, answer very well for the ventilation

Fig. 7.

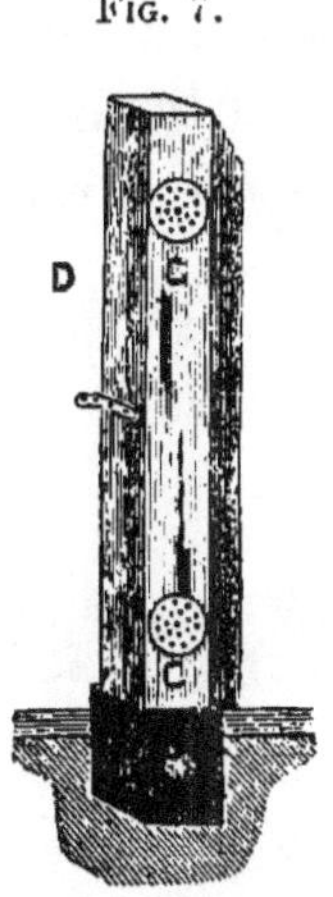

D. Wooden ventilating case. C C. Diffusion-openings.

of buildings already constructed, where there would be difficulty in carrying the diffusion-pipes up inside the masonry of the walls. They communicate with the barrack-flue, as shown in Fig. 8, and are provided at the proper intervals with exit-openings, in the same way as the diffusion-pipes.

Besides the diffusion-pipes in the side walls, or the side ventilating cases, two or more diffusion-cases must be erected in each barrack, according to its size. They should be twenty feet apart, and placed over the central flue, so as to receive air direct from it (o Figs. 2*a* and 8). They may be constructed of masonry or other strong materials, and should form ornamental tables; the interior consisting of a chamber having a measurement of 2ft. 3in. by 1ft. 4in. by 1ft. 2in., with openings at the four sides, similar to those in Fig. 4, c, for the exit of air; these openings must be of the same size as those in the walls and ventilating cases, and covered in the same way, with perforated zinc plates and iron gratings. Each chamber should have at the bottom a trap-door valve (Fig. 8, *a*) for the purpose of regulating the discharge of air.

Fig. 8.

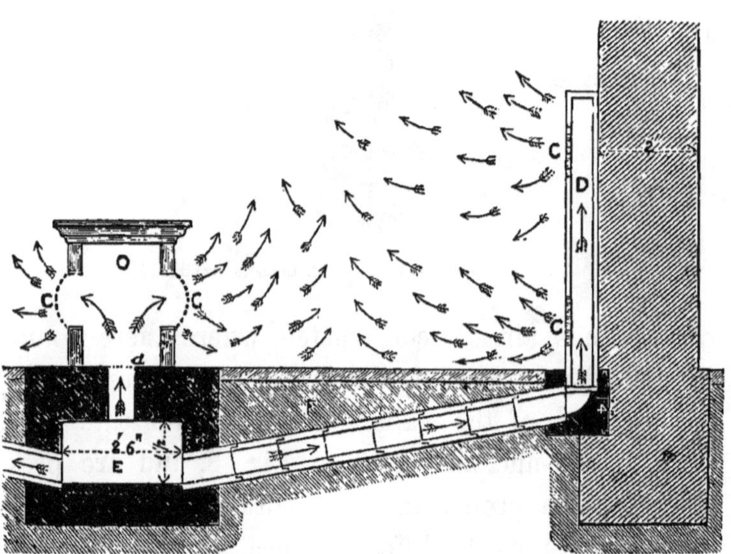

Sectional view of ventilating diffusion-apparatus, showing course of currents of air. C C. Exit-openings, covered with perforated metal. D. Ventilating case. E. Section of barrack-flue. F. Diffusion-pipe. O. Section of central diffusion-case. *a*. Trap-door valve.

The great object of these diffusion-cases being placed in the middle of the apartment is, that the air issuing from them on all sides shall, on meeting the currents from the openings in the walls, cause numerous eddies and other irregular movements in the air, and thus produce thorough ventilation of every corner of the barrack. (The various currents of entering air are represented by the arrows in Figs. 3, 4, and 8.) It has been estimated that, with the numerous openings, the ingress of air will be quite sufficient to supply at least 15 cubic feet to each man per minute —a quantity ample for all purposes. The volume of air, which should be completely changed in an apartment within a certain period, does not necessarily amount to the whole cubic capacity of that apartment; it is sufficient if it represents the cubic contents of the lower part, or that portion having for its area the length and breadth of the whole interior, and for its depth a little more than the height of a man, or, in round numbers, seven feet. This, in a barrack having a ground area of 200 feet by 20, is equal to 28,000 cubic feet—a quantity which the apparatus in question would renew completely, every fifteen or twenty minutes, in ten such barracks.

For the purpose of propelling the air, there are several different kinds of fans of excellent construction, any one of which would answer the purpose; but, of all that I have examined and seen at work, I would give the preference to Mr. George Lloyd's noiseless disc-fan (Figs. 9 and 10). The following is a description of the impeller, the case being much the same as that of most other fans. "It consists of a central boss, having around it several radial or curved arms, to which are bolted as many blades. These blades are of a tapering form, and are all arranged with their narrowest end outwards; to the side edges of the blades two circular conical-shaped metal-plates, of sufficient diameter to extend to their tips, are accurately fitted and fastened, the whole thus forming a hollow circular case, divided into compartments by the blades, with a central hole in each side, through which the fluid to be impelled is drawn, and an opening around its periphery, the same width as the tips of the blades. This arrange-

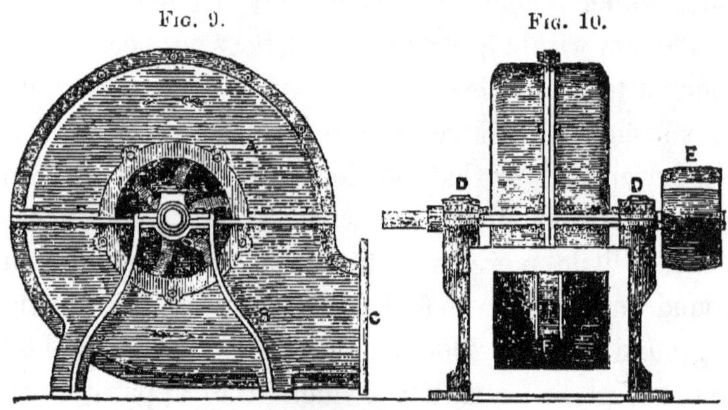

Lloyd's Noiseless Disc-Fan.

ment gvies a nearly uniform sectional space in any part of the impeller between the central holes and the periphery. The central boss is keyed firmly on a shaft passing through it, and on which it revolves on suitable bearings. In giving the impeller circular motion, the fluid is drawn in at the central holes, and discharged by centrifugal force, through the openings in the periphery, into the external case, whence it is forced through the discharge-pipe."

The following table gives the diameter of impeller, number of revolutions, and size of discharge-pipe, &c., of the fans made at present; but they can be constructed of any size.

The density of the blast is from a quarter of a pound to three pounds on the square inch.

These fans cost from £5 to £40 each, according to size; and a steam-engine, with boiler for wood fuel

Diameter of Impeller.	No. of Revolutions per Minute.	Horse-power required.	Diameter of Discharge-Pipe.	Cubic feet of Air per minute.*
13 inches.	1,800 to 2,000	½	5in. (round)	1,050
16 ,,	1,700 to 1,900	¾	6 ,,	1,500
19 ,,	1,600 to 1,800	1¼	8 ,,	1,750
22 ,,	1,500 to 1,700	2	9 ,,	2,000
25 ,,	1,400 to 1,600	2½	10 ,,	2,500
30 ,,	1,300 to 1.500	3	12 ,,	3,000
36 ,,	1,200 to 1,400	4	14 ,, (square)	5,000
42 ,,	1,000 to 1,200	5½	17 ,,	7,500
48 ,,	800 to 1,000	7	20 ,,	10,000

* These quantities are said to be considerably under the mark.

complete, of power sufficient to drive a pair of the largest-sized fans, would cost from £250 to £450 in this country. The same engine would, however, be available for other purposes, to be noticed hereafter; so that only a moiety of the expense would fall on the ventilation.

For the ventilation of barracks for the wing of a regiment, or any smaller number of men, where fans of a smaller size would be sufficient, American horse-tread mills, or the ordinary horse-power machinery, worked by bullocks (see Frontispiece), would answer as the motive power very well indeed; and for a still smaller number of men, the fans might be worked by hand.

In order that the air supplied to the barracks may be pure, and of even temperature, it should be drawn from a considerable height above the surface of the ground, say through a shaft or chimney, thirty or forty feet in height and six feet square inside, and so constructed that all communication with the ground can be effectually shut off.

Some years ago, I conducted a series of observations on the temperature of the atmosphere at night, at twenty-five feet from the ground, and found the range of the thermometer between sunset and sunrise very much less than within three feet of the earth, or even over the meteorological table, where the instruments were carefully protected from radiation. The register of these observations, which extended over about eighteen months, was destroyed in the mutiny in 1857; but I remember the evenness and comparatively less range of temperature, which I noted with considerable interest. I may mention, for the information of those who may wish to repeat the observations, that they were taken with two minimum thermometers and a long pole, placed in the middle of an open space, away from trees and buildings of all kinds. One of the thermometers was hung on the pole at three feet from the ground, and the other suspended at the top of it, by a cord which ran through a block and allowed the instrument to be lowered at pleasure for observation. The observations were taken regularly at sunset, 10 p.m., and sunrise. In addition to these observations, others were registered occasionally at shorter intervals. A moment's reflection will show any one possessed of ordinary meteorological knowledge, that the foregoing results were just what might be expected. At the same time, they are important facts, which, in addition to the other advantages of the supply of air for ventilation being drawn from a considerable height above the ground, should not be overlooked.

Means should also be provided for supplying the air cold or warm, as may be necessary. As the full propelling force of the fans should be available for driving the air to the extremities of the flues, it must be drawn, not forced, through the refrigerating or the heating apparatus.

For refrigeration, which will be more generally required in India than heating, the apartment H, Fig. 1, must be fitted with a series of "Khuss Tatties"* of sufficient extent to cool 20,000 cubic feet of air per minute from a temperature of 117°; for this purpose about 750 square feet of tattie will be required. If the cooling room be 23 ft. broad and 10 ft. in height, a tattie of this size would give a cooling surface of 250 square feet; so that three-inch tatties would, according to the above calculation, be sufficient; but for facility of renewal, repairs, &c., the tatties must be made in sections of about 25 square feet each part, and fitted into frame-work (Fig. 11, B), so that each large tattie would be composed of ten small ones of the above size (see Fig. 11). As a considerable portion of the dimensions of each tattie will be taken up by the frame-work, it will be necessary to have four rows, as shown in Figs. 4 and 11. The frames should be inclined at an angle of 25° or 30°, so as to afford greater facility of keeping the tatties wet. For this purpose inch-and-a-half water-pipes (Fig. 11, D)

---

* The *kus-kus* is a sweet-smelling grass, of which refrigerating "tatties or screens are made. In addition to cooling the air, the *kus-kus*, when kept moist, imparts to it a delicious aroma. When the temperature of the air outside stands at from 150° to 120° Fahr., that inside may, by the aid of these tatties, be kept at 80° or even lower.

should be laid under the floor of the cooling-room; and others, three-fourths of an inch in diameter, screwed on (Fig. 11, c) to these at right angles; the latter

FIG. 11.

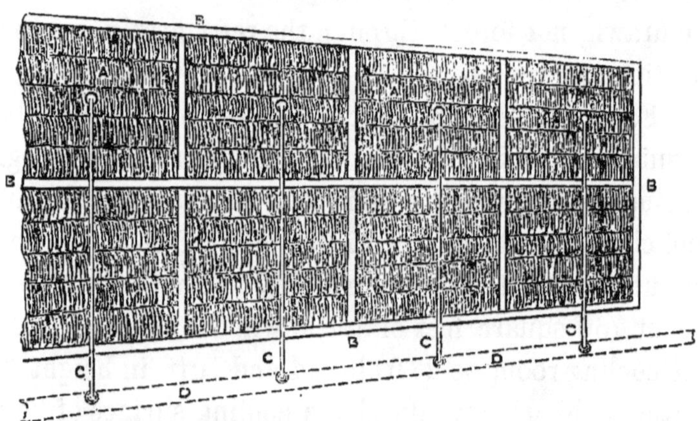

Part of a Khuss Tattie, or Refrigerating Screen, in position. B B B. Wooden frame, extending from side to side, and from top to bottom of cooling-room. C C C. Watering rods. D D. Water pipe underneath the floor of cooling-room, into which the watering rods are screwed when required.

must extend perpendicularly to within two feet of the top of the tatties. These perpendicular tubes must be perforated on the side facing the tatties, so as to throw a regular shower of water over a given space, say five feet in breadth and the whole height of the room, and thus provide thoroughly for the tatties being kept constantly wet without the aid of manual labour. Means for the supply of water will be described hereafter. An ice-making machine might be used for cooling the air; but a machine of the size that would be required would be very expensive; and, as the refrigeration is only required for a short time each year, the tatties, if properly arranged, will answer every purpose.

For warming purposes, nothing can be better than

hot-water pipes. In this case, three air-chambers will be necessary; namely, one for the hot-water pipes; one for the passage of cold air; and one for mixing the hot and cold air together (see Fig. 12). Whenever artificially warmed air is required—and it should always be used in the barracks at hill stations—the temperature should not be regulated by any interference with the hot-water pipes; they should always be maintained at an uniform heat, and the temperature of the air in the flues regulated by the admixture of cold air with the hot, as already described. This, if properly managed, will afford the means of maintaining the temperature of the air in the barracks to any required degree.

In addition to the other advantages of this system of ventilation, the air can be washed, by passing it through a shower of water impregnated with any of the permanganates or other disinfecting substance. The charcoal air-filter, described in my paper read before the British Association, could easily be brought into play in this mode of ventilation; but I believe that, if the air be drawn through a shaft forty feet in height, no filtering will be necessary.

All the egress-openings for the vitiated air should be in the roof, and should open direct into external space, so that the whole of the foul air may at once be carried clear away from the vicinity of the buildings. For an Indian climate, nothing can be better than open ridges, such as are in pretty general use at present; but they should be open from end to end of the building, so that there may be no obstruction to the direct ascent of the foul air.

Respired air invariably tends upwards at first, and

Fig. 12.

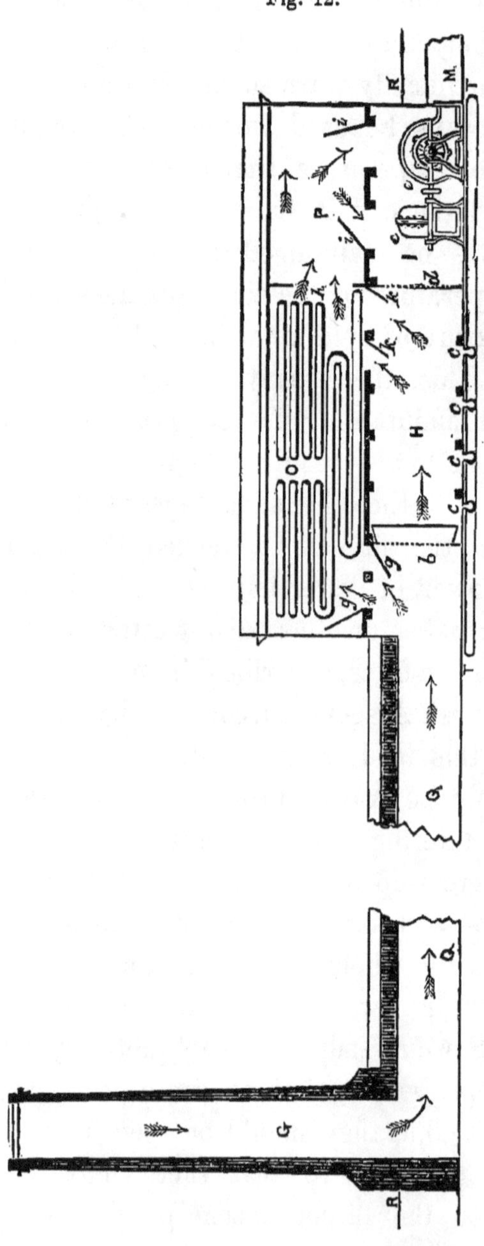

G. Fresh air-shaft. H. Refrigerating-room, without tatties and watering apparatus. I. Fan-room. M. Main flue O. Heating-room and apparatus. P. Mixing-room, for regulating the temperature of the air by the addition of the requisite quantity of cold air. R. Surface of the ground. T. Water-pipe. *b*. Valve for admission of fresh air to refrigerating-room. *c c*. Position of the tatties and watering rods. *d*. Valve for admission of cold air to fan-room. C. Fans. *g*. Valve for admission of fresh air to heating-room. *h*. Ditto to mixing-room. *i*. Valve for admission of warm air to fan-room. *k*. Valve for admission of cold air to mixing-room. The temperature of the air is regulated by the admission of cold air through *b* and *k*. When cold air only is required, valves *g*, *h*, *i*, and *k* are closed, and *b* and *d* opened.

thus, the ascending movement being its natural direction, it will be easily propelled onwards by a continuous stream of fresh air entering below; and, its place being thus occupied by a denser body, it can never again return to be re-inspired, provided proper arrangements have been made in the roof for its final exit.

The only objections to open ridges are the admission of dust during dust-storms, and of birds. The dust is a very trifling inconvenience in comparison with the advantages of free ventilation; and the birds, which are very troublesome and offensive, can easily be excluded by wire-netting fixed in framework, and fitted perpendicularly under the roof of the ridge. Galvanised wire-netting, with meshes sufficiently small to exclude small birds, costs about 2s. 6d. per square yard, so that the cost of such netting for a barrack 200 feet in length would amount to only about £30—a trifling outlay compared with the comfort of being free from such a nuisance.

Strong currents and draughts are arguments constantly urged against the "plenum method" of ventilation, but without good grounds, as I shall show hereafter. Other minor points, such as unequal action, choking of the flues with filth thrown into them, and so on, are so obviously easily provided against by the most ordinary care, that they hardly deserve notice. If the fans are worked by steam or other well-regulated motive power under proper control, the ventilation must be steady and uniform; much more so, indeed, than by any other means; and, the mouths of the diffusion-pipes being covered with finely-perforated plates, and protected by iron gratings to prevent injury to these plates, no filth can possibly enter the flues.

With reference to the strong currents and draughts alluded to, it must be borne in mind that the air will enter in fine jets, in oblique and horizontal directions, and is consequently easily deflected and readily diffused in the surrounding space, causing no perceptible draughts—at least no offensive ones—provided the renewed air be not at a very low temperature. Means have already been suggested for providing against this when necessary. It is evident that there can be no ventilation without movement of air; still, when this movement is duly regulated, according to the temperature of the air and the wants of the system, it is either altogether imperceptible or, at least, inoffensive. It is not the mere motion of air which is the cause of offence in draughts, but the movement of air in proportions or of a character uncongenial to the condition of the system at the moment. It has already been shown, that the due maintenance of health requires the body to be constantly surrounded with pure air; and that this can only be effected by the air being kept in constant circulation about the body, so as to carry off the noxious exhalations as they are formed. If the movement of the air be maintained at a steady pressure with no such sudden alterations of temperature as shall create an undue increase in evaporation from the surface of the body, no draughts will be felt, or, at least, no ill-effects will be experienced.

"The perfection of ventilation consists in the free supply of air, so completely attuned to and in harmony with the frame on which it acts, that its operation is not perceived;" and, as long as a certain relative uniformity of temperature is maintained steadily between the surface of the body and the surrounding air, this will be the case. It is on this principle that the punkah, so essential to health and comfort at certain seasons in India, acts beneficially. It does not change the air of the apartment or affect its temperature in the smallest degree; but it sets the atmosphere in motion, and thus enables a larger quantity to come into contact with the body in a given time. In this way there is established an increased and pretty uniform amount of evaporation of the perspiration, and consequently a reduction in temperature of the surface of the body generally, which renders a series of currents and draughts, so long as their action is steady and the temperature of the air moderate, highly agreeable to even delicate females, who would shudder at the mere mention of what is generally called a draught. This would lead to the inference, that a moderate current of air may be passed over the body with impunity—indeed, with decided advantage—under certain conditions, provided the temperature of the air be not very low, and the movement moderate and steady. In fact, we have familiar examples of this during the hot season in Upper India in almost every house, where every person who can afford it sits the whole day, and many sleep at night, with impunity, under the blast of a "thermantidote."

At lower temperatures, however, the case is different; as then, in addition to a certain amount of evaporation, there is a sudden abstraction of heat by the direct contact of the body with a cold fluid. The effect is consequently marked and disagreeable, or actually injurious, according to the rate at which the air moves.

In the plains of India, however, the temperature of the atmosphere very seldom falls so low as to be disagreeable, when the air moves in a very gentle continuous stream, so as not to be perceptible unless carefully noticed. This condition of matters, it is to be observed, would be fulfilled by the system here recommended. In the hills and other places, where the climate is to a certain extent cold for a few months of the year, the temperature of the air used in ventilation could very easily be regulated by artificial heat; but, with the exception of barracks at hill-stations, this would very rarely be necessary.

When ventilation would be required as a very temporary arrangement only, canvas tubes, of about the size, and made exactly on the principle of ship windsails, would answer the purpose very well. Some years ago I ventilated part of a house with common fanners and canvas tubes, and have since seen the air from an ordinary "thermantidote" conducted all over a large house by the same means. For the purpose under consideration, the main tube must, of course, be suspended horizontally along the middle of the barrack; and the diffusion-pipes must branch off at the proper places, in much the same way as the earthenware pipes from the underground flues. Though this apparatus is somewhat unsightly, compared to the more substantial plan of masonry flues, &c., it will effect perfect ventilation of every corner of an apartment.

The same system of ventilation applies, of course, to all places where large bodies of human beings are congregated together. In the case of prisons, where the fans are worked by the prisoners, it would not be convenient or advisable to have them outside the main wall; nor would it indeed be necessary, as the fans may be placed at any distance from the fresh-air shaft. The fans should be in the best position with relation to the cells and wards for forcing the fresh-air into them; and the fresh-air shaft should be in such a position as will insure a perfectly pure supply of air.

Ventilation of Tents.

The ventilation of tents, seeing that the cubic space per man is sometimes as low as 77 feet, never more than, and very rarely so much as, 220 feet, stands in even greater need of improvement than that of barracks. In the first place, the construction of the tents now in use is defective, inasmuch as they have not an opening round the pole in single-poled tents, and along the whole length of the ridge in double-poled tents, for the egress of the foul air. The remedy for this very great defect is so simple, that I think there must be tents with such openings, although I have never seen any of them. It merely consists in two feet of each fly round the pole in single poles, and on each side of the ridge in double poles, being made of strong rope lacing or net-work, instead of canvas, with a small canvas fly over all

Fig. 13.

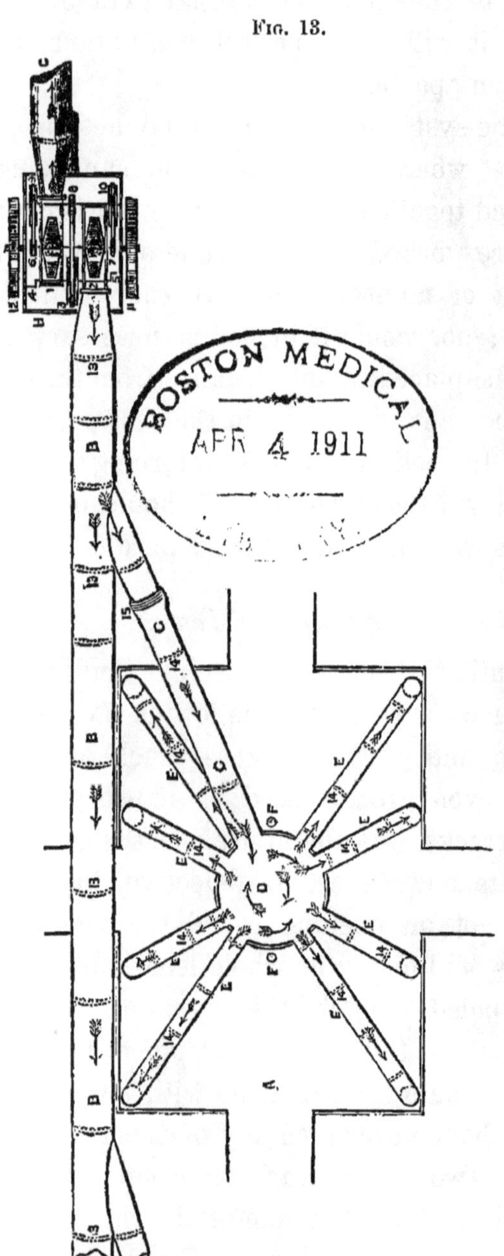

A. Ground plan of tent. B. Canvas main fresh-air tube. C. Tent fresh-air tube. D. Canvas diffusion-reservoir. E E. Canvas diffusion-pipes. F F. Tent-poles. G. Opposite canvas main, cut. H. Platform on wheels, with a pair of small 16-inch Lloyd's fans and driving gear. 1, 2. Small fans. 3. Driving wheel for fans. 4, 5. Crank for communicating motion to driving wheel. 6, 7. Pulleys on impeller shaft. 8, 9, 10. Duplicating gear. 11, 12. Wheels of carriage. 13, 13. Wooden distension-hoops of main tube. 14, 14. Wooden hoops for distending the tent-tubes and diffusion-pipes; all these being made of canvas. 15. Connecting joint.

(see Figs. 13 and 14), to keep out the wet. This will form a roof exactly like, in point of facility for ventilation, the roof with open ridge in barracks. Canvas so rapidly absorbs moisture, and along with it any impurities which may be suspended in it, that it is most desirable that the vitiated air, which is saturated with moisture, should be got rid of without remaining in contact with the cloth of the tent; and this will be readily effected, by its ascending direct into the open air through the openings round the poles and ridges.

As in the case of the barracks, however, open ridges without other means will not be sufficient for the ventilation of tents; and here again the plenum method, with fans, should be brought into play. One fan, with a sixteen-inch impeller, would be sufficient for the ventilation of accommodation for a company, or for one hundred individuals disposed in eight or ten tents. The fans (Fig. 13, 1 and 2; Fig. 14, M) should be arranged in pairs so as to propel the air in opposite directions, and placed so that one driving-wheel (Fig. 13, 3) will answer for both. The whole machinery should be firmly secured to a platform, and placed on wheels (Fig. 14, M), for the convenience of ready transport and action. The fans being small, the whole machinery of one pair, including the necessary appliances for the diffusion of the air for 200 individuals, would be a light load for one pair of bullocks, and consequently would always, during marches, be on the camping ground in time to commence the ventilation as soon as the tents were pitched. The fresh air would be conveyed from the fans to the tents in canvas tubes, and diffused in

Figs. 14, 15, 16.

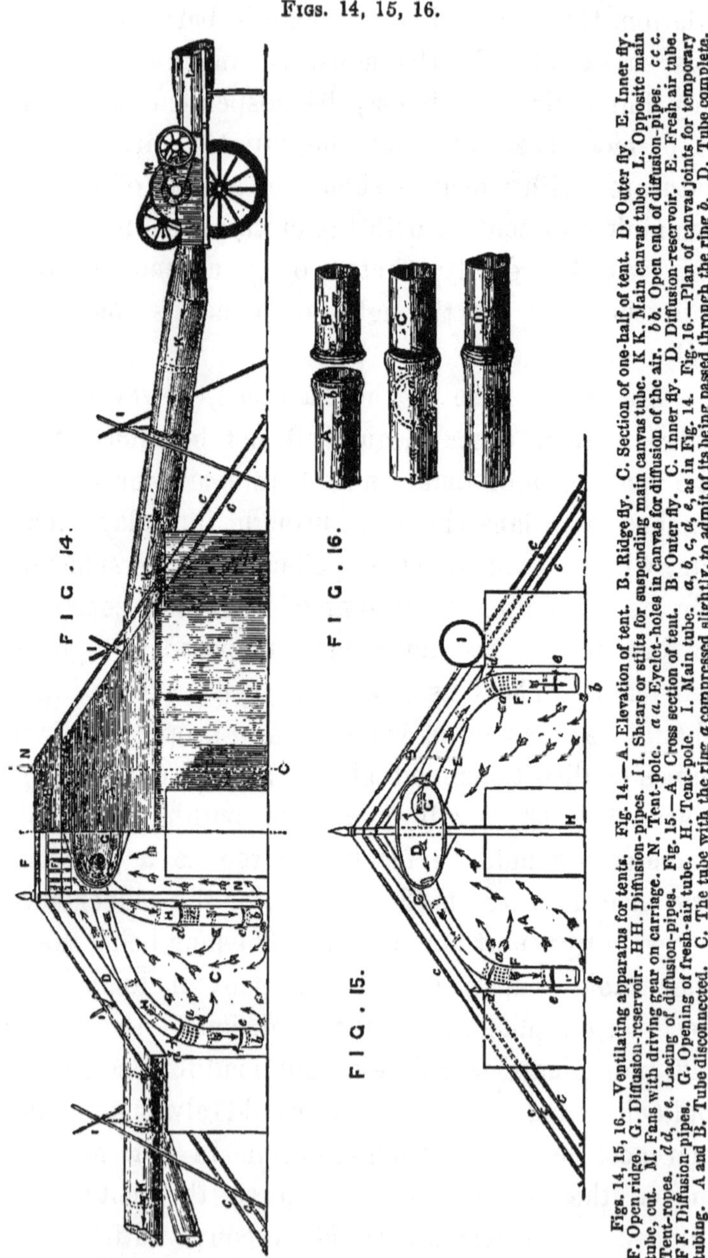

Figs. 14, 15, 16.—Ventilating apparatus for tents. Fig. 14.—A. Elevation of tent. B. Ridge fly. C. Section of one-half of tent. D. Outer fly. E. Inner fly. F. Open ridge. G. Diffusion-reservoir. H H. Diffusion-pipes. I I. Shears or stilts for suspending main canvas tube. K K. Main canvas tube. L. Opposite main tube, cut. M. Fans with driving gear on carriage. N. Tent-pole. *a a.* Eyelet-holes in canvas for diffusion of the air. *b b.* Open end of diffusion-pipes. *c c c.* Tent-ropes. *d d, e e.* Lacing of diffusion-pipes. Fig. 15.—A. Cross section of tent. B. Outer fly. C. Inner fly. D. Diffusion-reservoir. E. Fresh air tube. F F. Diffusion-pipes. G. Opening of fresh-air tube. H. Tent-pole. I. Main tube. *a, b, c, d, e,* as in Fig. 14. Fig. 16.—Plan of canvas joints for temporary tubing. A and B. Tube disconnected. C. The tube with the ring *a* compressed slightly, to admit of its being passed through the ring *b*. D. Tube complete.

very much the same way as suggested for the temporary ventilation of barracks. The main tube (Fig. 13, B; Fig. 14, K), made of canvas and wooden hoops, exactly like a ship's windsail, and of about the same diameter, should be carried along the windward side of the tents, on, or rather suspended from, light bamboo shears (Fig. 14). A branch tube for each tent (Fig. 13, C) will be sufficient.

If moderate care be observed in pitching the tents and placing the ventilating apparatus, the ventilation with canvas tubing will proceed in exactly the same way as in the more substantial masonry flues under ground. Supposing the tents which are to be ventilated are twenty in number, containing accommodation for two companies of European soldiers, the fans must be placed in the middle of the line, in such a position as to command as straight a course as possible in both directions for the main tubes B B and G (Fig. 13), which are suspended from bamboo shears or stilts (see I I I, Fig. 14) at a convenient height from the ground, and to windward of the tents when practicable. The air, being set in motion by the fans, will, as in the case of the permanent barracks, seek the most ready place of exit; and in doing so will enter the fresh air tubes (C, Fig. 13), pass on to the diffusion-reservoir D, and from it be diffused into the interior of the tent by the diffusion-pipes E E E (Fig. 13) and H H (Fig. 14). The foul air will make its escape through the open ridge of the tent at F.

In pitching the tents, it will be desirable to arrange them as regularly, and keep them as close together, as possible, as otherwise an unnecessary quantity of main tubing will be required. In other respects, no inconvenience can arise from irregularity in distance; as the fresh air supply-tube for each tent can be lengthened at will. The pitching of the tent being completed, the diffusing apparatus should next be adjusted by suspending the diffusion-reservoir to the ridge-pole, and securing it to the standard poles of the tent and loops on the inner fly and walls prepared for the purpose. The diffusion-pipes must be laced to the sides of the tent, near the eaves, and within about eighteen inches of the ground (see D D, and E E, Figs. 14 and 15); and lastly, the fresh air supply-tube, being passed through the opening made for it between the wall and fly in the end of the tent, will be joined to the main by a joint at 15, Fig. 13. The fresh air will escape from the diffusion-pipes, through eyelet-holes, a little below the eaves of the tent, and at the lower ends of the tubes. (See A A, and B B, Figs. 14 and 15).

A few words regarding the management of the connecting-joint, which, as far as I know, is quite new, may be useful. The ring *a* (Fig. 16) is a very little longer than the ring *b*; but by compressing it a very little it takes an oval shape, and readily passes through the latter; and, the pressure being withdrawn, it immediately assumes its circular form, and catches behind the ring *b*. Traction being made on B, the tube takes the connected form D. A few pieces of tube, with connecting-joint ends, should always be kept at hand. With a pair of spare stilts and a short piece of tube, with joint-ends, no real difficulty can arise in adjusting the apparatus, as by these means the distance between any two given points can be increased or decreased at pleasure.

Fans of the size already described discharge 1,500 cubic feet of air per minute, and cost at the foundry £7. A pair of such fans, with driving gear, platform, and carriage complete, would probably cost 500 rupees by the time the apparatus could be ready for use, exclusive of tubing, which could be procured in India.

It must be borne in mind that, while men quartered in tents continue to sleep on the ground, no system of ventilation, however perfect, can render the atmosphere pure and healthy; but this, like the other defects in tents, might very easily be remedied. Instead of the clumsy uncomfortable wooden bedsteads supplied at present for the use of European soldiers in India, why should they not have folding iron ones, which, in ordinary times of peace, they would always carry with them, and for the safety and good order of which they should be held responsible, in the same manner as for any other part of their kit? I have seen several kinds of folding iron bedsteads, admirably suited for the purpose in question. These bedsteads weigh about 52lbs., and, I believe, could be supplied of a strong substantial description for from 15 to 18 shillings each. There are such articles as low as 7s. 6d.; but the more expensive ones, being stronger and better made, would be cheaper in the end.

The carriage of all these additional necessaries will probably be objected to; and, as a matter of course, additional carriage would be necessary on their account; but in times of peace troops are not constantly on the move, and in ordinary marches sixteen carts would be sufficient for the conveyance of the ventilating apparatus and bedsteads of a whole regiment of a thousand strong.

Ventilation on the "Plenum" Principle. St. George's Hall.

For ventilation on the "plenum" or impulsive principle, preference is generally given, both in this country and in America, to large fans, of from ten to twenty feet in diameter, revolving at a slow speed of about fifty or sixty revolutions per minute. No doubt they answer admirably where one building only has to be ventilated, and where the basement story is available for the machinery, so as to obviate the necessity of forcing the air through flues of any great length.

Were it necessary to discuss further the advantages of this method, many excellent examples of ventilation with fans of various constructions and sizes, &c., all more or less effective, could be cited. A few words on one of them, however, may not be out of place; namely, St. George's Hall, Liverpool, the ventilation of which was executed under the direction and supervision of the late Dr. Boswell Reid, who ventilated several other public buildings on the plenum principle, and very justly stood high as an authority on questions of ventilation. In the ventilation of this building there are four large fans, each ten feet in diameter, driven by a steam-engine, and making from fifty to sixty revolutions per minute. They are placed about the centre of the building, in the basement floor. Three fans impel the fresh air through a series of large horizontal flues or passages, into which the greater part of the basement is divided; and it is finally diffused into the great hall, courts, and other apartments, through trellised work and openings in the sides of the floors and wall, most of which are covered with gratings. The flues are fitted with valves, which are, in reality, large folding doors, arranged in every conceivable position likely to be useful in giving the air every required direction, and for affording the ready admixture of heated air with the cold atmosphere. By this means a uniform temperature of about 60 Fahr., or any other required degree, can be maintained for any length of time all over the building. The vitiated air escapes through numerous openings about the cornices and ornamental open work in the ceiling, into a large air-chamber between the arched roof of the great hall and the outer roof of the building, and finally passes through a large shaft into the open air. The foul air vents and shaft are provided with gas-burners, for the purpose of creating a draught through; but I was informed that it was very seldom found necessary to light these burners. The ventilation of this very large building appears to be as complete as could possibly be desired. On the occasion of my last visit the sessions were being held, and consequently all the courts were crowded, and there were great numbers of people all over the place, yet the air was perfectly free from all unpleasant smell. The temperature in the court room was 66°, and not the least draught was perceptible in any part of it.

To ventilate barracks on an extensive scale with large fans, placed in the position recommended by Dr. Reid, would be an extremely expensive matter; and unnecessarily so, seeing that the same results can be obtained with smaller fans revolving at a greater speed. To reach the extremities of comparatively small flues of great length, the air must necessarily leave the mouth of the fan at a considerable velocity and pressure; but it does not follow that there must be offensive currents in the apartments ventilated. On the contrary, if proper attention is paid to the perforated coverings of the openings for the exit of air, imperceptible diffusion can be effected, at least as much so as when the motion of the air is slow and the openings for its diffusion are large.

CHAPTER III.

WATER.

It has been estimated that more than 70 per cent. of all living organic matter consists of water; and, as this large proportion is obtained, in one way or another, from the food and liquids taken into the stomach, it will be at once evident that the greatest care is called for, in providing it for domestic purposes, that it be of a pure and wholesome quality.

Chemistry of Water.

Water, which was considered an elementary substance by the old philosophers, is composed of hydrogen and oxygen, in the proportions of two measures of the former to one of the latter by volume, or one part of hydrogen to eight of oxygen by weight; that is, the union of these two gases in these proportions produces water. It is, however, never found absolutely pure in any quantity. In nature, it always holds in solution or suspension a variety of substances more or less beneficial or injurious in the animal economy, according to the nature of the substance and to the condition of the body at the time when it is received into the system. Water, as it is met with in nature, contains always more or less of saline and mineral matters, in proportions varying with the nature and composition of the soil and rocks over which it flows or through which it percolates; and, in addition to "these inorganic substances, it contains organic matters arising from the decomposition of animal and vegetable substances, either growing in the water or cast into it."

In all countries, water for domestic purposes is procured from much the same kind of sources, namely, running streams, surface-wells, tanks, and deep wells; and contains silica, salts of potash, soda, magnesia, lime, organic matter, and sometimes other substances in certain proportions, according to the composition of the soil of the locality, and the depth of the wells from which it is obtained. As far as these specialities are concerned, the quantities of organic and inorganic matters in water will bear a certain relative proportion in every country where the soil is of alluvial formation. But it must be borne in mind that, in addition to their natural composition, all soils near the surface of the earth contain more or less of the substances thrown on the ground, and that surface-water is very liable to hold in solution or suspension substances which do not belong to the soil naturally, and may be very local in their origin. As the composition of the water of few localities has been more carefully determined than in that of London, the following comparative statement of the quantities of organic and inorganic matters in some of the waters supplied to London and its neighbourhood will illustrate the large quantity of foreign substances which water may hold in solution or suspension, and show, in some degree, what may be expected in water supplied for domestic purposes in India, where it is chiefly obtained from surface-wells and tanks.

	Organic matter.	Inorganic matter.	Total.	Analyst.
SURFACE WELLS.	Grains per gal.	Grains per gal.		
Belgrave-mews	15	110	125	Aldis.
Grafton-street.................	26	115	141	Hillier.
Wandsworth-road	19	72	91	Odling.
Spencer's-court	14	172	186	R. D. Thomson.
Broad-street, Golden-square.	5	102	107	Powell.
RIVER WATER.				
Grand Junction Water Company	1·5	21·5	23·5	Hoffman.
New River	1	21·0	22·0	"
Thames, at Twickenham ...	2	20·0	22·0	Clark.
DEEP WELLS IN CHALK.				
Trafalgar-square	...	68·00	68·00	Abel.
Richmond	·80	27·20	28·00	Henry.
Long-acre	...	57·00	57·00	Graham.*

From the above analyses, it will be seen that the water of surface-wells contains by far the largest quantity of organic matter—a circumstance which must invariably be the case wherever the wells derive their supply from the percolation of moisture through the subsoil, or from water flowing directly into them from the surface of the ground.

Water-Supply in India.

Although many of the wells in India are very deep, in some cases upwards of 150 feet, still the average is under 40 feet; and the whole water-supply is from the surface in some shape or other. If filtration through the subsoil be not sufficient to purify the water of the organic matters taken up in

* Dr. E. Lankester's "Guide to the Food Collection of the South Kensington Museum."

its first contact with the earth, it will, in a great proportion of cases, become impure; and, the water being sparkling and to all appearance pure, from the carbonic acid generated in the course of the decomposition of the organic matter and more or less saline matter held in solution in the water, the impurity will escape detection. However, it so happens that the subsoil is, as a general rule, quite sufficient to purify the water as it passes through it; and it issues at the bottom of wells 25 or 30 feet deep sufficiently free of organic matter to render it quite pure enough for all ordinary purposes. It always contains more or less of inorganic substances, such as some of the salts of potash, carbonate of soda, chloride of sodium, and carbonate and sulphate of lime, but in such small quantities as to be inappreciable, or, at least, harmless in their effects. Wherever it is otherwise, the taste will discover the injurious excess, and the evil will be avoided.

But, although organic impurities do not enter the wells and tanks from below, a sufficient quantity does reach them by direct means, in many instances, to render the water supplied for domestic purposes in India often absolutely filthy. When a native bathes he does not carry the water to a distance from the well for the purpose, but he sits on the edge of it, and pours the water over his body, allowing it to run back into the well; and he not only washes his body in this way, but also any little clothes he may have about him, which must be saturated with perspiration and other filth. Hence every well frequented by natives, and the ground immediately round it, contains a great deal of the organic matter daily given off by two or three hundred human beings. Again, tanks are, if possible, worse; for, if the bathers do not go into them bodily, every drop of water, as it runs off them and is wrung from their wet clothes, returns into the tank. Who, that has seen a large encampment, can have escaped remarking the lively scenes at the wells and tanks in the vicinity at night, although he may have overlooked the fact that his cup of tea the following morning will be prepared with a portion of the water he has just seen used in washing the bodies and clothes of fifty dirty human beings?

With regard to rivers, no description can convey an idea of their filthy state, particularly in the lower parts of the country. In addition to all other kinds of filth, the dead are thrown into the rivers, instead of being burnt or interred; and thousands are disposed of in this way annually. I have myself seen upwards of fifty dead human bodies, besides numbers of carcases of lower animals, floating in the River Hooghly, within sight at one time; and these corpses float up and down with the tide until the flesh falls off the bones, and they sink to the bottom, or lie exposed, at low water, on the muddy banks.

Impurity of Wells.

It is by no means determined that all impurities in wells emanate solely from either of the sources already indicated. It must be borne in mind that these wells, which supply the chief part of the water used for domestic purposes, stand constantly open-mouthed, ready to receive everything that may come their way. Is it not, then, very probable that some, at present undetermined, deleterious substances are swept into them by the wind? and are they not very likely receptacles for a subtle, invisible poison, like that of malaria, which always hangs near the earth in low situations, and of which we at present know little or nothing, except that, the closer to the ground its victims are situated, the more sure is its action, and the more fatal its result?

We know also that foul air will accumulate in any well, however pure the water *per se* may be; and, as water absorbs gases rapidly, if left in contact with foul air it very soon becomes highly impure, particularly on the surface. It is therefore evident that the use of water that has remained stagnant for even only a few days in deep wells should be avoided. But, instead of this, the only means of supplying water for domestic purposes in India, provides that the most impure water of every well shall be first used. When a person on a march arrives at the end of his day's journey, his water-carrier proceeds to the nearest well, and with a small leathern bucket draws water for his use, which must necessarily be from the very surface of the well, for he has not the means of drawing it from the bottom; and consequently the water supplied is more or less impure, according to the time it has remained stagnant, to say nothing of the other sources of impurities already noticed. The same thing takes place with regiments or small parties of men marching through the country. The men arrive, at the end of the day's march, tired and thirsty, and the first thing they do is to gulp down a draught of water procured from the surface of the nearest well, which has remained stagnant, it may be, for weeks. Again, on the arrival of troops at new stations, the water first used has very often been stagnant in the wells for considerable periods; so that whole regiments may, and indeed do, often use for months continuously water charged with malarious organic poisons, without being in the least degree aware of it, for in taste, and to all appearance, the water may be pure and sweet.

However, let the impurities and their source be what they may, we have too good reason to know that they do exist, and that they are more or less obnoxious to health according to circumstances. Hence the necessity for a plentiful supply of pure water for the troops is a matter of the first importance; and this can very easily be effected with ordinary care, and at no very great additional expense to that attending the present very defective system.

Provision of Pure Water.

In the first place, the supply should be plentiful, and drawn from near the bottom of deep wells; and in the second, all the water used for drinking and culinary purposes, whether in cantonments or on the march, should be properly filtered.

It is very rarely the case that pure water, at least sufficiently so for all ordinary domestic purposes, cannot be obtained by digging deeply enough for it; and, therefore, wherever the water is brackish or otherwise impure, the boring should be continued until strata bearing sweet water are reached. At places such as Agra and Cawnpore, for instance, where the water in some of the wells is sweet and in others brackish, there can be little doubt that, by boring deeply enough, say within two hundred feet, sweet water could be procured at almost any point. In fact, at the former place, the wells from which the best water is obtained are all very deep; and, as these wells are not confined to one particular part, but are found in uncertain localities in and about the station, it may fairly be assumed that the strata bearing sweet water extend under the whole area of the district, and could be reached within a reasonable depth; and this would, no doubt, be the case at all the other stations in India, where brackish water exists in impure wells.

For the supply of a regiment, say one thousand strong, in cantonments, one well, with two sets of pumps and one filter, would be quite sufficient. The well should be in the vicinity of the ventilating apparatus (Fig. 1, p. 31); so that the same steam-engine would answer for driving the fans, pumps, and ice-making machine. The filter may be situated either at the well or at any other convenient place. Cheap and efficient filters could very easily be erected at the barracks; but water absorbs gases so rapidly, that it should never be stored in any quantity near places where it might be exposed to foul air. If the filter be distant from the well, the only difference will be the cost of additional pipe for conveying the water from the well to it. There are many excellent kinds of pumps, each claiming its own special advantages; but I would recommend the one called the

California lift, a diagram and description of which will be given under the head of Water Supply for Camp (p. 71). It is very simple, least likely to get out of order, and the most economical of all the pumps I have seen at work. It will answer for any depth of well, from ten to upwards of two hundred feet, and can be worked either by hand, steam, or other power. It can be made of any size; but a pair of small pumps will be better than one large one, for the reason that repairs can be effected without discontinuing the supply of water, and the first cost will not be much more than that of one large one. Two five-inch cylinder pumps will raise 5,200 gallons per hour, or 62,400 in twelve hours, equal to fifty gallons per man *per diem*, for upwards of 1200 men; a quantity more than sufficient for every purpose for a whole regiment, including swimming baths, irrigation of gardens, &c.

The filter may be constructed of either iron or masonry; and the plan represented in Fig. 17 (p. 68) will be found easily arranged, efficient, and economical.

Water-pipes should be laid on to each barrack, in the usual way, so as to afford a ready and plentiful supply of water at all times, without the aid of water-carriers, who should be completely dispensed with. Attached to each barrack should be one or more drinking fountains; and none can be better for the purpose than those manufactured by Messrs. Macfarlane and Co., of Glasgow. These fountains have self-acting spring stop-cocks, and consequently prevent the possibility of unnecessary wastage from leaving the cocks open. They are very neat, clean, take up little space, and are cheap. Fountains like

FIG. 17.

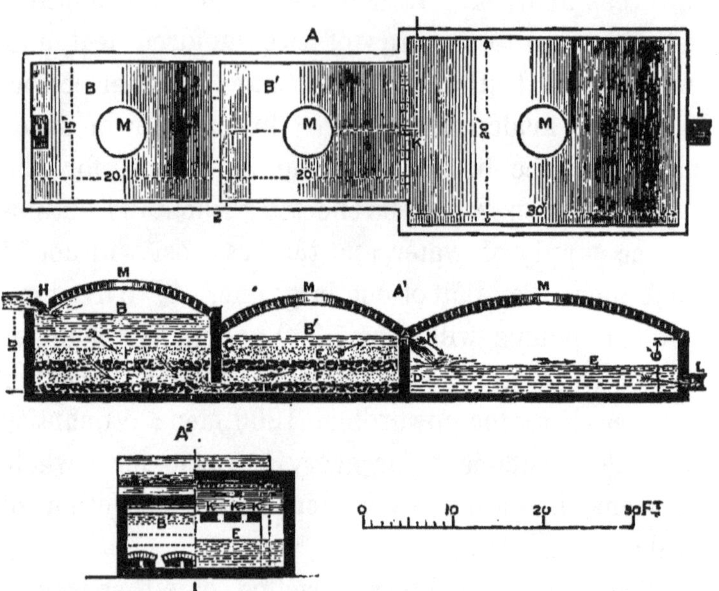

Filter for Barracks. A. Ground plan. A1 Longitudinal section. A2 Cross section. B. Unfiltered water. B1 Filtered water. C. Diaphragm of filter. D. Separation wall between filter and reservoir. E. Reservoir for filtered water. F F. Gravel and fine sand (15 inches). G. Charcoal (15 inches). H. Feed-hole. I. Passage under diaphragm of filter, for water in process of filtration. K K. Passage for filtered water into reservoir. L. Distribution-pipe. M M. Man-holes for gaining admission into filtered reservoir. These man-holes should be kept carefully closed, except when absolutely required to be open for cleaning or repairing the interior of the apparatus.

the sketch Fig. 18* would answer admirably for the purpose, and should be unsparingly supplied. Amongst their many advantages, they will obviate the necessity for drinking water that has lain long in dirty vessels; and they will go far in preventing the men from having recourse to the grog-bottle. If a glass of pure cold water were always available, there

* One of this description costs at the foundry £2 18s. 6d.

would be far less inducement for indulging in ardent spirits. It is all very well to preach against the abuse of spirits—and it cannot be too severely

Fig. 18.

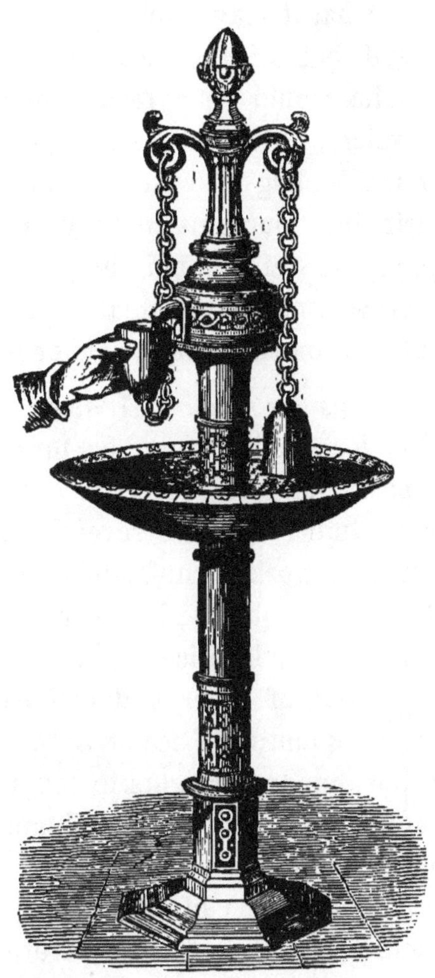

Drinking Fountain.

deprecated--but, with nothing better than a little dirty warm water to drink, in a dry, hot, sultry night, when a person is parched with thirst to the last degree, there are few who could resist the temptation of mixing a little spirits with such beverage. Warm water and rum are more palatable, at any time, than stale warm water by itself. Let the reason be what it may, tippling only requires a beginning; and one of the best preventives, particularly in India, would be a ready supply of pure fresh, cold water. Were a cistern properly constructed for the cooling of water by ice connected with the drinking fountains already described, a supply of good cold water would always be available, and would prove one of the greatest boons which could be conferred on the British soldier in India.

Means for Cooling Water.

The means for cooling water or for other refrigerating purposes, need no longer be a desideratum in any part of India. I have several times lately seen a machine at work manufacturing ice of great density and excellent quality, in every respect quite as good as any river or lake ice. These machines do not readily get out of order, and can be made to manufacture any quantity of ice at a very moderate cost, from a few hundred-weights to ten tons daily; so that an unlimited supply can be obtained at any place, no matter what the temperature of the atmosphere may be. On each of the occasions when I saw the machine at work, the temperature in the refrigerating cylinder was below zero Fahr., and the apparatus usually worked at 10° below this point.*

* This machine was invented by Mr. James Taylor, of Messrs. James Taylor and Co., No. 13, Fenchurch-buildings, London, who is always most obliging in showing one of the machines at work. The machines can be turned out complete at from £60 to £300 each, according to size.

The machine is so constructed, that any increase in the temperature of the surrounding atmosphere or water used for condensation, &c., is compensated by a proportionate increase in the motive power which drives the machine. Wherever these machines are used, two small ones would be preferable to a single large one, as then, in the event of anything going wrong with one of them, the supply of ice would not be interrupted. The machine should of course be placed near the ventilating apparatus, as shown in Fig 1 (page 31).

Water-Supply for Camp.

With reference to the supply of pure water for troops on the march, the means are not quite so simple; but still, with ordinary care, it can easily be effected. It has been already stated that the water in deep wells, which are not constantly used, is very liable to become impure, particularly on the surface; and that, on account of the present mode of drawing water from wells in India, this foul surface-water is unavoidably always the first used. To remedy this serious evil, two or more wells should be fitted with pumps, on the principle of the California lift (Fig. 19), which, being partly suction and partly force, will answer for any depth, and can be fixed in existing wells without any alterations, with the exception of a beam being let into the old masonry. Four different sizes of these pumps, which lift from 500 to 2,000 gallons in an hour, can be worked by hand, and consequently are particularly well adapted for the purpose under consideration.

Supposing the surface of the water in a well in which one of these pumps is to be fixed to be fifty feet from the surface of the ground, a beam, L, Fig. 19, must be let into the masonry, A, of the well, say

Fig. 19.

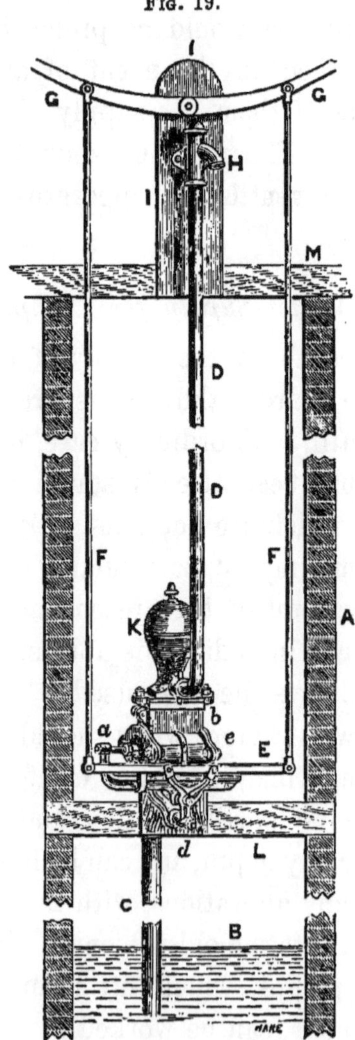

California lift pump. A. Masonry of well. B. Surface of water. C. Suction-pipe. DD. Force-pipe. E, F, G. Levers. H. Discharge spout. I. Piece of wood to which head of force-pipe is fixed. K. Pump. L. Bar for supporting Pump. M. Edge of well. *a.* Sliding bar. *b d.* Rocking arm. *e.* Cylinder.

twelve or fifteen feet above the surface of the water. To this beam the pump, K, must be bolted, the suction-pipe, G, being sufficiently long to reach within about a foot or so of the bottom of the well, and the force-pipe, D, sufficiently long to admit of the discharge-spout, H, being about four feet above the edge of the well. A strong piece of wood, I, must be secured in a perpendicular position to the edge of the well, M, and to it the head, H, of the force-pipe, and the lever, G, must be bolted. When the lever, G, is raised or depressed, it imparts motion through the bar, F, to the lever, E, which in turn communicates it to the rocking arm, *d*, and from it to the sliding bar, *a*, which is attached to the piston in the interior of the cylinder, *e*; and thus the whole apparatus of the pump is set in motion. Pumps with three-inch cylinders would be the most convenient in size for the purpose in question, and the most economical in first outlay*.

For the filtration of water in camp, Atkins's Moulded Carbon Filters are peculiarly adapted; they can be moved from place to place without the least chance of drainage or interference with their action in any way. They are constructed of galvanised wrought-iron tanks, with moveable water-tight covers, and man- and feeding-holes in the top. Each tank has one or more patent filters securely fastened in it, so as to prevent oscillation or breakage, with discharge-pipes fitted with stop-cocks projecting through the tank, and affording ready access to the filtered

* Hand-pumps, with cylinders three inches in diameter, cost £5 each at the factory.

water. They have also air- and water-plugs, and every means for cleaning and keeping them in good order. The filters are made of perforated earthenware or galvanised wrought-iron cylinders, covered with horse-hair cloth. Each cylinder has a series of moulded carbon blocks, through which the water percolates into the discharge-pipes; and, in addition to these blocks, the cylinders are packed full with pieces of charcoal, so that as far as filtration by charcoal goes the process is as perfect as could be desired. These filters are said not only to clarify the water by arresting the mechanical impurities, but to purify it by causing the oxidation of organic matter. I have seen them in use, both in my own house and in other places, and can speak most favourably of their action and usefulness.

Tanks measuring 3ft. 6in. by 2ft. 6in. by 2ft. 6in.

Fig. 20.

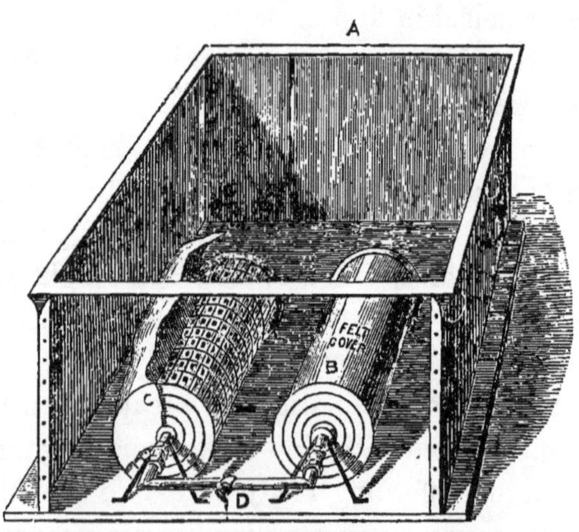

A. Tank with two filters. B. Filter with felt covering. C. Filter with covering turned back. D. Self-acting spring stop-cock.

would hold about 120 gallons, with two filters (see Fig. 20), which would weigh, when full, about fifteen hundred-weight, or say 21 maunds, and filter between 300 and 400 gallons *per diem*. This would be a very convenient size. I have suggested to the makers the advantage of such filters for certain purposes being mounted on spring-carriages, as represented in Fig. 21, and they are prepared to

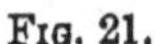

Fig. 21.

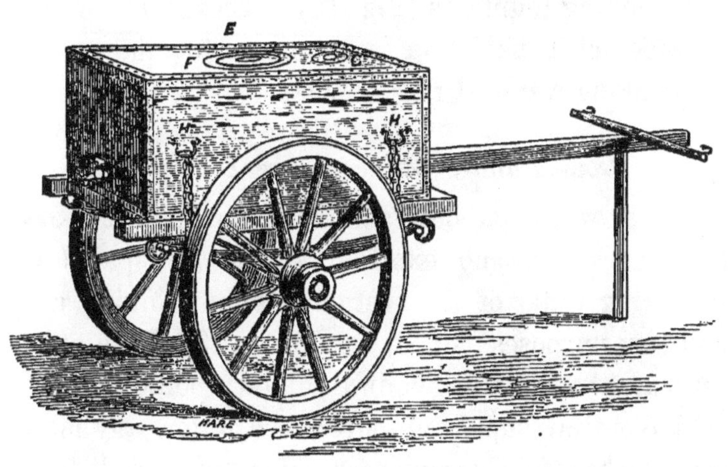

E. Filter on spring bullock-truck. D. Self-acting spring stop-cock. F. Man-hole. G. Feed-hole. H H. Handles for lifting the filter and securing it to the truck.

guarantee the action of the filters so arranged. In fact, I have had one shaken about in every possible way likely to disarrange its parts, without producing any damaging effect on its action.

With a sufficient number of these filters, say one of the dimensions specified above to every two companies, the men need never, on any occasion, be without a plentiful supply of pure sweet water. Even during the march, a certain number of the tanks should always be kept within convenient distance of the column, so as to completely obviate the necessity of the men ever having recourse to the water-carrier's dirty "mussak," not always supplied with even the best water available; and in camp they should be arranged in fixed localities, so that every man may know where to look for a glass of pure sweet water. To prevent wastage the filters should be fitted with self-acting spring stop-cocks (D), as recommended for the drinking fountains (Fig. 18). These tanks would also be most useful in cantonments for the supply of drinking water at the barracks.

Does Impure Water cause Disease?

After what has been said, it is hardly necessary to remark that no exertion should be spared in procuring water of the best quality for drinking and culinary purposes; for it would be difficult to overestimate the advantages, in a sanitary point of view, of a plentiful supply of pure fresh water, any more than the baneful consequences which must result from the use of bad meat, bread, or any other impure or bad article of diet. But I consider that, however necessary it is to pay strict attention to the quality of the water, undue importance is very often attached to impure water as a primary source of disease, and that the real cause—namely, foul air—is overlooked. I would venture to predict that, as sanitary science advances, this view of the question will be established.

As water springs from the interior of the earth, where its source cannot be examined, so that a fair field for any amount of speculation exists regarding substances which cannot readily be clearly determined, but which we generally know to exist in some shape, any broad assertion that impurities in the water are the cause of some peculiar epidemic is readily received without question, and very often forms a convenient way of accounting for some unusual state of things which might not be easily disposed of in any other way.

We not unfrequently find that some sudden outbreak of disease is attributed to "something in the water," without attempting to define what that something is; and with no better grounds for saying so, than that there is something in the bread or meat; except that impurities in water are not so easily detected, and no one is responsible for what the earth supplies, it being taken for granted that better cannot be procured. This is, however, a mistake. Pure air and water are, under proper arrangements, as procurable as any of the other necessaries of life; and there ought to be an authority attached to every department and regiment, as responsible for the quantity and quality of the water supplied to the troops, as the commissariat is for the bread and meat; and until it is so, the men will not be so healthy as they might be.

But, to return to the subject of water not being always such a ready and fertile source of disease as is generally supposed; everyone who has seen the Hooghly must have been struck with the intensely dirty state of the river. In addition to the sewage of the town of Calcutta and the other towns and villages on the banks of the river, thousands of dead bodies and carcases of dead animals float about in it, until the flesh is completely decomposed and the bones fall to the bottom; yet we have no positive proof that the water is injurious to health to the extent some authorities would wish us to believe. Were it so, few of the ships which arrive at Calcutta would ever leave it again; for nine-tenths of the crews would be poisoned by the water. From the day a ship arrives at Calcutta until it leaves again—indeed, until, the homeward voyage is half and sometimes wholly completed—the crew is supplied entirely with Hooghly water, which is not always filtered. But, under the most favourable circumstances, it is only filtered from the river alongside the ship by passing through a small filter, in the entire charge of natives, as rapidly as a pair of force-pumps can send it into casks on board; that is, at about the rate of 500 gallons per hour.* During the time a ship lies at Calcutta, this said filter-boat goes alongside periodically, and pumps in a small supply of water for the daily use of the crew; but a common practice is simply to allow the water drawn direct from the river to stand in tubs until the mud and other mechanical impurities subside, when it is considered fit for use. And there cannot be much difference between water clarified in this way and the so-called filtered water, seeing the rate at which it passes through the filter.

* I have myself seen, more than once, a dead body hanging across the bows of the filter-boat, without any attempt being made to remove it by the people in charge of the boat.

Notwithstanding all the sources of impurities referred to, and the opinions which have been occasionally advanced regarding Hooghly water being the cause of cholera and other diseases on board ship, it is generally considered good; and the Fort William Special Committee considered it sufficiently so to recommend a steam-pump for the purpose of supplying the Fort with water for all purposes. In one of the special reports relating to Fort William at Calcutta, submitted to the Royal Commission on the Sanitary State of the Army in India, it is stated that, "The river being unsuitable for six weeks annually, masonry tanks within the Fort have been recommended, having stowage space for two months' supply of pure water for drinking and culinary purposes, the quantity so stored to be calculated at one cubic foot per head *per diem*."

"The following table shows the chemical analysis of the Hooghly river water from off Fort Point, on the 30th April, 1860, at low water, by Dr. Macnamara, Professor of Chemistry:—

Silica	0·5
Earthy carbonates	2·5
Sulphate of lime	0·3
Alkaline sulphates	1·1
Common salt	4·1
Alkaline carbonates, and a little soluble organic matter	0·9
Solid residue from 40 ounces.	9·4

"The water was filtered before analysis; but, the river being unusually low at the time the water was taken, its impurities were probably at the maximum. The water is soft, and its quality is good and not injurious to health."*

It has been stated that cholera, which prevailed on board ship on one or two occasions in the Bay of Bengal, was caused by the use of Hooghly water; but I think such an opinion must have been given at random. I was long connected with ships trading to Calcutta, and was intimately acquainted with the captains and officers in the same service; and never once heard of the cholera breaking out on board in an epidemic form after the ship was fairly at sea. I believe that if it ever do so, it must be more from over-crowding and something very defective in the ventilation and cleanliness of the ship, than from any other cause.

I made ten voyages to Calcutta, and had medical charge of four different detachments of European invalids from that place to England, and never saw any disease among the troops, crew, or passengers, which I could attribute to bad water. I always found my treatment successful, perhaps more so at sea than I could have always expected on shore; and generally found the cause of anxiety to diminish the longer we were at sea, even with regard to cases of chronic bowel-complaints (very common amongst all Indian invalids). This could have hardly been the case if the water had any influence, seeing that impure water is generally considered a fruitful source

* Royal Commission on the Sanitary State of the Army in India. Vol. ii., page 11.

of acute diseases of this kind. The only conclusions that can be drawn from these facts are, either that the Hooghly water was sufficiently pure for drinking and culinary purposes, or that filthy water very seldom has the bad effects generally imputed to it.

During our stay in Calcutta, we had occasionally a great deal of cholera among the sailors; but, from a great proportion of the cases occurring on the second day after the men returned from being on liberty, it struck me that the disease had been contracted in some way on shore. On two occasions, there were a few cases among the troops during the first three days after they embarked, in consequence, apparently, of previous dissipation. I never had a fatal case among the officers of the ship, nor met with the disease among the passengers; and never had a case after the ship was fairly at sea. This happy state of things could hardly have existed for such a long period, had the Hooghly water been a very fruitful source of the disease. It is to be observed (and I think deserves some attention) that I always belonged to large, well-ventilated ships, where every attention was paid to cleanliness and comfort; but the water was from the river, as with any other ship.

Were careful inquiry instituted, I believe it would be found that, in every instance where cholera has made its appearance, or fever or any other epidemic has prevailed on board ship, they could be traced to some other cause than impurities in the water. We have well-authenticated instances of cholera being confined to a particular side of a ship, and the officers and other groups of individuals on board having marked immunity from the disease, which could hardly be the case if the water were the cause of mischief among the rest of the crew. An instance is given by Dr. R. D. Thomson, in his evidence before the India Army Sanitary Commission, in which he attributes an outbreak of cholera on board a ship, of which he was in medical charge at Bombay, to impure water. The men, however, who were attacked with the disease, had been working in the ship's hold, where the atmosphere was very close and hot, and there was an abominable stink from part of the cargo, consisting of decomposing sharks' fins; and the cholera disappeared in three days after the men were prevented from working in the hold, while the shore-men, who continued the stowing of the cargo, were reported to have died of cholera after they went on shore.* Here

* "I may mention another case in which I consider water was connected with cholera. On arriving at Bombay, 12th May, it was reported that no cases of cholera existed in the town. The temperature was then at 80°, and the wind westerly, with a clear sky. On the 15th the disease appeared in the town. Cases of cholera were frequent on board ship in the harbour about the 24th. The first case of cholera occurred on the 7th June, and terminated fatally. The wind was now south-westerly, and the monsoon being about to set in, which it did on the 14th, with rain. On the 8th two cases of cholera occurred; on the 15th there was another case of cholera, and on the 16th a fatal case. These men had been working in the hold, and using Bombay water. In the hold the heat and closeness were very great, and the abominable odour of sharks' fins, part of the cargo, was very annoying. The portion of the hold where the men had been stowing cotton, I found, extinguished a Davy lamp. From this period no Europeans were allowed to stow; and on the 18th they were replaced by Seedies, powerful Muscat men. Cholera disappeared from the ship. The Seedies worked for some days and then left for the shore, and were reported to have died of cholera. The water of Bombay I found to contain much organic matter, having been taken from a tank * * * * * These waters contain much organic matter in solution; a considerable amount in suspension, and common salt, sulphate and carbonate of lime."—Dr. R. D. Thomson, in Minute of Evidence taken before the Commissioners appointed to Inquire into the Sanitary State of the Army in India, page 274.

is an instructive case, where the water is found, by an accomplished chemist, to contain a large quantity of organic matter; but the history of the progress of the disease does not bear out the impure-water theory. The sailors who were attacked with the disease were employed in the ship's hold, which was teeming with foul air sufficient to extinguish a Davy lamp. The disease disappeared in a remarkably short time after those affected were prevented from working in this foul atmosphere; and the strong healthy men from the shore, who took their place in this same foul air, were reported to have died of the disease from which the sailors had suffered while they inhaled it—a very natural result of such a state of things.

Instances of this kind might be enumerated to almost any extent. I remember a ship lying in the Hooghly, directly opposite the Fort-ditch, the crew of which were suffering severely from cholera. It was suggested that the water might be the cause; but, as other water could not be procured, the next best thing was to move the ship away from the vicinity of the filthy ditch, which had the happiest effect, the disease disappearing almost immediately. The ship was moved about five hundred yards from the original position, further down the river; and if there were anything peculiarly more filthy in the water of the ditch than in the river (which was hardly possible), the ship was more in its way than at first. Possibly the water said to have been the cause of disease on board ship, may have been taken from the river during the season when it is considered "unsuitable for culinary and drinking purposes;" but after what has been shown to be the state of the river all the year round, it is difficult to believe that the water can be pure at any season.*

If we turn again to the Prison Returns of the North-West Provinces, where the water has been obtained from the same wells ever since the jails were in existence, and must be the same always (except when the number of prisoners is in excess, when it will to a certain extent be fresher on account of a larger quantity being drawn), we shall find a marked immunity from cholera among the prisoners, except in jails where they are overcrowded. Here the disease proves as virulent as in any other place where large numbers of human beings are massed together in confined spaces.

In the report of the commissioners appointed to inquire into the Epidemic Cholera of 1861 in Northern India, much valuable information will be found on the subject of impure water; and they seem to have arrived at the conclusion "that mere contamination of the drinking water may cause disease but will not cause cholera."†

---

* Any one wishing to peruse this part of the subject further will find all the information he can possibly require in an able paper on the mortality of Calcutta, by Dr. Hugh Macpherson, in the "Indian Annals of Medical Science," 1862.

† "Much has been said in Europe regarding the propagation of cholera by impure drinking water, and the evidence that has been produced to show that it has in some cases happened, appears so strong that it is hardly possible to dispute it. Here, again, we seem to find a repetition of the facts upon which we have before laid stress. In the same manner that no atmospheric condition, and no local sanitary conditions appear to be alone capable of producing cholera, so it seems with impure water. Nothing could be worse than the water supply of some places in England which escaped the attack of cholera, while the disease was raging in the neighbourhood. Mere contamination of the drinking

Although it is not the object of this treatise to discuss the various theories of the sources of cholera, it may not be out of place to remark here that we may, and often do, find cholera where the water used for domestic purposes is perfectly pure, but we very rarely meet with the disease in an epidemic form where there is not good reason to suspect the existence of foul air at the time of the outbreak of the disease, or shortly before it. Again, whatever may be the ultimate effect of impure water on the system, we know that it may be continued for a long time, when even highly charged with impurities without producing any serious consequences. (See what has already been said regarding the use of Hooghly water.) But no person can live in foul air, if in any excess, for even a short period, without the most serious results ensuing. However, when both impure air and water are in operation at the same time, which very often happens, and was the case at Mean Meer in 1861, the consequences cannot fail in being most serious. If cholera do not ensue, some other disease of almost as fatal a nature is sure to be propagated. In addition to all the other sources of foul air enumerated by the Commissioners appointed to inquire into the matter, 1,500 men were located, at Mean Meer, in buildings barely sufficient for 1,000,*

water may cause disease, but it will not cause cholera. The specific poison must in this case also be present."—Report of the Commissioners appointed to Inquire into the Cholera Epidemic of 1861 in Northern India.

* "The buildings, both barracks and hospital, which were intended for one regiment, and were not complete even for this strength, were occupied at the outbreak of the epidemic, not only by a full regiment H. M.'s 51st, but by the right wing of H. M.'s 94th regiment also. Thus, more than 1500 men were placed in buildings barely sufficient for the proper accommodation of 1000.

and the water of several of the wells from which the troops were supplied contained, according to the analysis of Dr. Brown, chemical examiner at Lahore, a very large quantity of organic matter and other impurities.

No one, however much impressed with the conviction that impure water will not, as it is usually met with in the wells, tanks, and rivers in India *per se*, produce cholera, will dispute for a moment the fact that bad water, like other articles of diet of an inferior or bad quality, if continued for any length of time, must lower the tone of the general health, and in this way aid considerably in the propagation of diseases such as bowel-complaints, and it may be, under certain conditions, cholera and dysentery; and therefore, as already stated, every possible care should be taken to insure that the water supplied for drinking and culinary purposes is of the best quality; but the influence of impure water *per se*, as an active agent in the production of disease, if it merely contain organic matter in solution, is not so great as is generally supposed. If water, however, contain inorganic substances, such as sulphate and carbonate of soda, chloride of sodium, sulphate and carbonate of magnesia, nitrates of potash and soda, &c., which it frequently does, derived from the early geological formations and soil through which it percolates, and

Each barrack, which could only properly hold 96 men, was occupied by 115. * * * * * It became necessary to place men in the inner verandahs, for there was no other means of accommodating them; and such an arrangement seriously interferes with the ventilation of the main rooms. In buildings constructed on the plan of these barracks, overcrowding ought especially to be avoided. Under any circumstances their proper ventilation is difficult, on account of the numerous inner walls and subdivisions of rooms and verandahs."—Report of the Commissioners appointed to Inquire into the Cholera Epidemic of 1861 in Northern India.

sometimes, particularly in the case of some nitrates, formed from the oxidation of ammonia, derived from recent animal matters in the soil of certain localities, the case will be different, and the water will then act as an active poison. All well-water, although it may be to all appearance perfectly pure and sparkling, contains more or less saline matter, the nature of the salts varying with the character of the soil through which the water percolates; but any competent chemist will always be able to detect these impurities; and, when they exist in unusual excess, the water should of course be carefully avoided.

No one would think of purchasing a bag of flour or a piece of meat without first examining them, and ascertaining whether they were of good quality, and sufficient in every way for the purpose for which they were intended. If a contractor supplies bad food, it is at once rejected. The same care should be extended to the supply of water; and, whenever there is the least doubt regarding its purity, its composition should be carefully ascertained by chemical analysis, and rejected if impure.

The greatest evil with regard to water in India is, after all, the scanty supply. Now there is no good reason for this. Water can be procured in any quantity by digging for it; and with good pumps and a good steam-engine, or bullock-power properly managed (a very simple matter), there is no difficulty in bringing water to the surface; when it is there, the filtration and distribution of it in the usual way, as already explained, is simply a matter of first expense, but true economy in the end.

CHAPTER IV.

FOOD.

To discuss the properties of the various kinds of food as fully as the subject deserves, would far exceed the space that can be devoted to the whole question of sanitary improvement in a short practical treatise of this kind. As, moreover, a great part of the diet of the British soldier in India—consisting of meat, 1 lb.; bread, 1 lb.; vegetables, 1 lb.; rice, 4 ozs.; sugar, $2\frac{1}{2}$ ozs.; tea or coffee, $1\frac{3}{4}$ ozs., salt, 1 oz.; and firewoood, 3 lbs. daily—has been pronounced by high authorities to be generally good, I shall confine my remarks to a few practical hints on the most prominent points which require attention, and which may be improved without interfering materially with existing arrangements.

Quantity and Quality.

The diet supplied by Government is, perhaps, more faulty in being too liberal than in any other respect; for it is now well known that the quantity of food in a tropical climate is much more frequently to blame than the quality, in causing impaired health, such as disease of the liver, dysentery, diarrhœa, and other complaints usually attributed to the climate. Sir J. R. Martin, than whom no better authority could be cited, states that "an attention to quantity is of infinitely more consequence than the quality of our repasts, and that a due regulation of this important matter will turn out a powerful engine in the preservation of health.*"

The most abstemious are the most healthy men in India. In fact, no change that has lately taken place in the habits of the European residents has contributed more to health, than the discontinuance of heavy luncheons at one or two o'clock, so universal at one time, and the reduction of meat, in the bill of fare of the better classes, to one meal daily. Some people still take "tiffin" as amusement—perhaps the most expensive amusement that could be indulged in; but fortunately it is now generally confined to a little bread and butter and fruit, with perhaps a glass of wine. It would be well if the soldiers' diet could be reduced in the same degree to some equally simple fare, except, perhaps, during four months of the cold season, when they are actively engaged in duty or amusement out of doors. Indeed, the reduction might be made all the year round; for meat once a day—namely, at the principal meal, say about 2 o'clock p.m.—is quite sufficient, as far as this article of diet goes, for the support of the body in a state of strength and vigour. The classes from whom the most robust recruits are enlisted never have meat more than once a day, and not always so often; and the average quantity of food daily consumed by each individual does not amount to the allowance of a soldier by

* "The Influence of Tropical Climates," by Sir J. R. Martin, page 127.

several ounces; yet the labour they perform is very much heavier. What, then, can be the necessity for this liberal allowance, which all admit to be absolutely injurious, particularly in a tropical climate? However, "in order to have strong and brave soldiers, they must be well fed;" and therefore the total amount of ration should not be reduced, but the constituents of it should be carefully regulated according to the season and other circumstances, and strict care should be taken that they be suitably prepared, and not spoiled in the cooking.

In lieu of a portion of the meat, dall, one of the best articles of diet for a hot climate, with the usual condiments for cooking with it, should be allowed, and varied, on alternate days, with dried fruits, such as raisins, apricots, plums, dates, &c., which can be procured in India of excellent quality, and might be stewed, made into light puddings and dumplings, or eaten in the dried state, and form an agreeable addition to the dietary. If these articles were constituted a portion of the diet scale, regularly served out on fixed days, and properly prepared by the cooks, they would form a very useful change; and no doubt the men would soon prefer them to the never varying routine of meat.

Importance of Vegetables. Gardens.

One, or indeed I may say the greatest defect in the diet of the European soldier, is the want of a due amount of vegetables. If the want of a plentiful supply of this most essential article of diet is the cause of disease in other groups of individuals, why should it not be equally so amongst soldiers? In fact, they are often so badly supplied with vegetables, that there can be no doubt that dysentery, diarrhœa, and other complaints which very often assume a scorbutic character, may in a great measure be attributed to this cause.

The two principal difficulties connected with the supply of good fresh vegetables for troops are, the cultivation of them in the first instance, and the inducing the men to use them after they have been procured—a point which is by no means so easy as might be supposed.* About two years ago, an application was made to the Prison Department relating to the supply of vegetables for the troops from jail gardens, which led to some inquiries being made regarding the probable quantity that would be required, and the probability or otherwise of the vegetables being thrown on the hands of the Department after they were cultivated. The result was not encouraging, and I presume the Military Department found their inquiries unsatisfactory; at least, the question never took a practical form, which it might easily have done by securing the Prison Department against loss. How-

* There is an anecdote told of an application having been made not long ago to an officer in charge of the public garden, at one of the large stations in the North-West Provinces, for vegetables for the troops. He happened to have at the time a quantity of very fine vegetables, grown from English seed, of which he was rather proud; and to make sure that they were delivered in good order he went himself to the barracks, and was not a little disappointed to find that the men would not look at his fine vegetables. Some of them selected a few of the best of the cauliflowers; and others said they might accept a few good fresh peas if they were shelled. This was most probably an extreme case, and the men may have refused the vegetables from knowing that they could not get them properly cooked.

ever, if barrack-gardens were established on a proper footing, the first difficulty would disappear; and the second would be rendered much more simple, as the men would take more readily to vegetables cultivated by themselves. A plentiful supply being always at hand, there could be no excuse on the score of quantity; and their use should be compulsory. Moreover, there is a wide difference between a salad or any other vegetable fresh from the garden, and one that has been half the day in a dirty, smoky cook-house, after having been carried some miles in a dry wind or in a hot sun.

The proper cooking of vegetables is one of the nice points in the art, which, most likely, is not always found among the qualifications of barrack-cooks; but, if the means be afforded them, they can and ought to be taught; for the very best vegetable, like other articles of diet, may be rendered useless in the cooking. However, this cannot affect the use of salads and fruit, which, whenever procurable, should form a part of every person's daily food. "The consumption of a few ounces of uncooked fruit, such as pears, apples, oranges, grapes, &c., and, when these cannot be got, the various plants eaten as salads, is, I believe, essential to the diet of those who would maintain their health in perfect integrity."*

With regard to the gardens and their cultivation, I would offer a few remarks. The gardens should belong to barracks, and not to regiments, and the men occupying the barracks should simply be encou-

* "Popular Lectures on Food," by E. Lankester, M.D., page 58.

raged as much as possible to cultivate them, by receiving a moderate allowance per maund for the produce actually cultivated by themselves. Horticultural shows and prizes should also be established. If neglected, especially in the matter of irrigation, a garden will become a barren waste in an almost incredibly short time,* therefore these gardens should not be left entirely in the hands of the soldiers, who are frequently changing from one station to another. A gardener ("Malee") should be attached to each garden, who would be responsible for the proper irrigation of the soil at all times, and for the cultivation of the whole garden while the barracks remained empty on any occasion, and during the time that the new occupants might require to settle down into regular habits.

Meat. Parasitic Disease.

A great deal of the meat used by common soldiers in India, more particularly that portion of it procured for them at their own cost in the bazaar by the mess-cooks, is of the very worst kind. The bacon and pork, of which they are very fond and of which they eat freely, is badly and most filthily fed; "the bazaar pigs are the bazaar scavengers," and the flesh of them, when kept for even a very short time,

---

* On the day the mutiny broke out at Allygurh my garden was in a high state of cultivation, and in as flourishing a condition as could be wished. When I visited it again, just eight days afterwards, the leaves had all fallen off, the fruit-trees and everything were dried up, and so damaged for want of water, that the two years during which I remained at the place after the restoration of order were not sufficient to restore the garden to its former state of fertility.

actually smells of the very filth on which they had been living.

Our present knowledge of parasitic complaints conveys only a very limited idea of the diseases produced by parasites in the living body; but from the researches of Professor Owen, Mr. Paget, Professors Virchow and Zenker, M. Davaine, and others, they evidently exist to a very much more alarming extent than is supposed. In a paper by Mr. John Gamgee,* of Edinburgh, published lately in the

* "There are those who fancy that domesticity breeds disease—that improving the meat-producing powers and hastening the growth of our live stock, renders it liable to disorder of a malignant type. No greater fallacy! The parasitic maladies which are bred for man in the systems of the animals which we eat, are most common in the quadrupeds allowed to rove about in search of food, and which, living amongst men and animals, have every opportunity of meeting with the germs of the worms which prey upon them.

"In the pig, thousands of trichinæ may exist without affecting the animal's health; though commonly at the period of migration from the alimentary canal to the muscular system, there are diarrhœa, lassitude, and a general feverish state. These symptoms may be so severe as to kill, or may pass off; and either the animal lives on with trichinæ in the flesh, which afterwards die and cretify, or within a fortnight or a month there is evidence of pain, stiffness in movements, languor, debility, and death.

"What we see in the lower animals has been witnessed in man; and cases are accumulating so as to teach physicians how to diagnose the trichinæ in the living subject.

"Professor Zenker, of Dresden, mentions that among 136 *post-mortem* examinations which he made during eight months, in the year 1856, he found four subjects evidently afflicted with trichinæ. He gives the case of a farm girl who died under his observation in 1860, killed by trichinæ. She had, a month before, been taking part with the other farm-servants in a particular pig-sticking and in the consequent processes; and had probably (according to what is said to be not a very unusual practice) an occasional pinch of the sausage-meat which she had to chop. She soon fell ill, and died in a few weeks. Her bowels contained swarms of adult trichinæ, and the voluntary muscles throughout her entire body were colonised by myriads of larvæ. It appeared on inquiry, that other persons who took part in slaughtering the same pig also suffered; and that, though none died, two were bed-ridden for weeks. Micro-

"Popular Science Review," he gives some very interesting information regarding the existence of parasitic worms, more particularly the *Trichina spiralis*, in the flesh of pigs and other animals, which are communicated to human beings by the flesh of these animals used as food. Sheep and goats, when not sufficiently fed, eat ordure and other kinds of filth readily, and their flesh often contains parasites and several kinds of larger worms in great numbers; the rot and sturdy, diseases generally confined to sheep, but found in other animals, are parasitic diseases,* which may exist for some time without the animals affected with them exhibiting any marked signs, at least to the ordinary observer, of being out of health.

If the viands on the table of the officer or private gentleman, who pays a high price for them, be of indifferent quality, which they generally are when his servant has a contract for these supplies, what must be the case with the table of the common soldier, who contracts with a public servant for perhaps as great a variety for a mere trifle, and whose first object is quantity, not quality? Whether the meat is diseased or not, the articles of diet supplied on contract by soldiers' cooks are not likely to be of

---

scopical examination of products which were remaining of that of the slaughtered pig—ham, sausages, and black puddings, showed in them innumerable dead larvæ. Similar instances are recorded in this country."—"Popular Science Review," January, 1864.

* The Fluke (*Distoma hepaticum*) is generally met with in the liver, sometimes in great numbers. It is a flat, thin animal, about three-quarters of an inch in length, and half an inch in breadth. Sturdy (*Hydatis polycephalus cerebralis*) is considered to be worms in a particular stage of development.—McGillivray's "Veterinary Manual."

very good quality; and the practice should be put a stop to, as far as possible, by issuing all small supplies procured in this way from Government stores or regimental clubs at fixed rates; and, were properly conducted dairies and stock farms established in the vicinity of all military stations, the other extra articles, such as butter, eggs, milk, fowls, &c., could be procured of the best quality at a moderate cost.*

Cooking Arrangements.

Food, good enough in the first instance, is often spoiled in the cooking; and, notwithstanding the ingenuity of Indian cooks, it could hardly be otherwise in cooking on a large scale with the appliances at their disposal. Let the quality of the cooked food in nutritive elements be what it may, the mode of cooking and the cook-rooms are most defective, and in many instances filthy to a degree. The preparation of the food is usually conducted on a dirty mat, spread on the floor of the cook-house, the luxury of a clean dresser or table for the purpose being rare. What, then, must be the consequence, on a hot day, of the cooks and others employed bending over the food, as

---

* I laid before Government, some time ago, a scheme for the establishment of a convict farm at each of the large stations in the North-West Provinces, namely, Benares, Allahabad, Agra, Meerut, and Bareilly. This, if ever carried into effect, would not only supply at these places a great part of the articles alluded to above, but pave the way for the introduction of a better system of agriculture, horticulture, and the management of stock in the country generally. In all these there is very great room for improvement, development, and augmentation. It is said, and with good reason, that stock, such as cattle and sheep, are diminishing at an alarming rapidity, both in quantity and in quality.

well as other sources of filth, which need not be described, to say nothing of the swarms of flies, which are a most fruitful source of contamination to every article of food they touch? What may not be the bad consequences, in a kitchen, of a swarm of "blue-bottle" flies direct from the dead-house of a hospital? These are, perhaps, extreme evils, but they do exist, and ought to be looked in the face.

The cook-rooms, instead of being well lighted and properly defended from flies, external dust, and dirt, are dirty, smoky places, open to every filth that may be blown their way, generally without proper furniture and tables for dressing the food on, and with no better arrangement for the supply of water than what is afforded by the "Bhestie's mussak" and a few open earthen jars, seldom or never cleaned out, and generally used until they fall to pieces, which fortunately is very often. Parties may be told off to superintend the cooking, but they could not exist in such places in the hot weather for even half the time required to cook a dinner.

The cook-rooms should be large, airy apartments, well lighted and ventilated, carefully defended from the flies, external dust, and dirt; they should have a plentiful supply of water laid on in iron pipes; they should be liberally supplied with suitable furniture, particularly strong, substantial tables for dressing the meat on; and one end of the kitchen should be fitted up as a larder, the openings of which should be covered with wire-cloth, to exclude the flies. In lieu of the present defective system, a proper cooking apparatus should be introduced into every kitchen.* There can be no reason against the introduction of proper cooking ranges and appliances in India; on the contrary, their general application would be most useful and economical.

If the cook-rooms, which should be ventilated on the principle recommended for barracks in the first part of this treatise, were large, well lighted, comfortable places, head cooks could be selected from among the men themselves to superintend the cooking; and the whole process would be conducted in a cleanly, efficient manner, which would add immensely to the comfort and health of the troops.

The barrack cook-rooms are not the only places of the same kind in India which require attention. In fact, a clean, well-arranged kitchen might almost be considered the exception; for it is to be feared that the cook-rooms of all classes, which ought to be amongst the cleanest, are not unfrequently the dirtiest places on the whole premises, and are, no doubt, a fruitful source of disease in many instances. This may be startling, but it is nevertheless perfectly true. Our kitchens generally look clean and nice when visited; but are proper measures always taken to provide against their being occupied at night, particularly in the cold season? and are they not very often crowded with the cook's friends, gossiping over a friendly pipe, at the very time when he is

* The cooking apparatus described at page 107 of the Report of the Commission appointed for Improving the Sanitary Condition of Barracks and Hospitals, or, indeed, several of the many other excellent plans in use at large public establishments in England, would answer admirably for India.

preparing his master's principal meal? and is care always taken to see that the water, which has been standing by the side of these tenants of the kitchen for hours, is duly replaced by a fresh supply in the morning, before the cook commences his daily avocations? These, as well as many other sanitary arrangements, which demand constant attention in all countries, particularly where servants are not over-given to cleanliness, are, I fear, neglected; and, doubtless, many pay dearly for their neglect. But I have said enough to be a warning to those who fear paying a visit to the kitchen, lest they should see some filthy proceeding which would disgust them and prevent their enjoying the anticipated meal.

CHAPTER V.

CONSERVANCY.

There is nothing that calls more urgently for improvement in India than conservancy. The whole country, in this respect, may be said to stand very much in the same condition in which it was a hundred and more years ago. A great deal has been done lately in the depuration of military stations and some of the large towns, but the very difficult question of systematic conservancy may be considered still in its infancy throughout India. On account of the peculiar habits of the people, which, in most respects, are dirty in the extreme, amendment in the conservancy of a great portion of native towns is almost hopeless, and, under the most favourable circumstances, must necessarily be a very gradual process; but, with regard to the towns and villages in the vicinity of and adjoining European stations, immediate improvement should be strictly enforced. Efficient conservancy is simply a matter of expense; a circumstance not peculiar to India, for efficient conservancy is in all countries the largest item in municipal expenditure.

Several plans of improving the conservancy of military cantonments, jails, and other public places in India, and eve the native towns, have been tried with a certain degree of usefulness; but all fall far short of the desired efficiency. What is called the "dry system," which has always been the mode of disposing of the night-soil and sweepings of private dwellings, and which has been for a number of years* in operation on a large scale in some of the jails, is no doubt the best that has hitherto been adopted; but, even when carried out with great care, under the best supervision, such a system must be, at least, very defective.

The efficient working of a complicated system of conservancy of this kind, however good in principle, depends on too many individuals, particularly a class of men whom nothing but the greatest vigilance in unremitting European supervision can keep at their work. This vigilance cannot always be employed in full force, especially in the hot weather, and therefore the proper working of the system must be at the lowest ebb at the very time when it ought to be in the most active and perfect operation; namely, at the season when organic matters of all kinds run into a putrefactive state with the greatest rapidity. Moreover, there can be no reason for continuing a complicated system, the efficiency of which must at all times be

---

* As far back as 1845, the late Mr. William Woodcock, of the Civil Service, then Inspector of Prisons in the North West Provinces, discontinued, in the jails under his care, the use of drains for carrying off the sewage, and introduced the system of the removal by hand of all night-soil, sweepings, and filth of every kind, to a distance from the jails. He insisted on the use of heaps of dry sand under and around the night-urinals for the temporary absorption of any urine that might escape past the vessels, with excellent effect. He also introduced the frequent washing of the floors and walls of the wards with clay—a sanitary measure deserving more attention, I believe, than it has hitherto received.

more or less at the mercy of careless, idle servants, when a simple, effectual, and economical plan is available, which will not only provide for perfect conservancy, but turn the sewage to useful account at the same time—a matter of no minor importance in an economical point of view, as the value of the sewage as manure must eventually more than cover the expense of working the whole system.

Independently of excrementitious matter becoming rapidly putrescent, particularly in a hot climate, it gives off impure gases from the moment it comes into contact with the atmosphere. Moreover, the excreta of human beings who are not very careful about their food, even in point of quantity, are seldom quite healthy; and we know that the first dawn of approaching ill-health will generally be found in the altered condition of the alvine discharges and urine. In the first stages of some, and perhaps all, epidemics, one of the earliest signs, were these matters always carefully examined, would in all probability be found in some decidedly unhealthy change in the alvine discharges. At all events, in the most formidable of these diseases—namely, cholera and dysentery—the first well-marked symptoms show themselves in the frequency and unnatural condition of the evacuations; and it not unfrequently happens that those symptoms continue for some time before a person feels seriously ill, so that the excreta of nearly a whole regiment or other large body of individuals may be in a putrid, or at least semi-putrid state, giving off most dangerous gases for days before it is considered necessary to separate those affected from the main group. I believe that the part which the excrementitious matters of the affected play in the dissemination of epidemic disease, is chiefly due to the gases given off by them immediately or soon after they are voided, which gases enter the system through the lungs; and that, as already stated, the disease is communicated in this way, and rarely through the stomach. Let this be as it may, no one will deny the danger of inhaling these gases. How necessary, then, does it become that they should be fixed as quickly as possible, and thereby be prevented from being diffused among the healthy—a most desirable end, which, under the best possible arrangements, can only be very partially effected by the "dry system." The introduction, however, of carbolic acid* as a disinfectant and antiseptic, has completely supplied this great desideratum in conservancy; and now, by mixture or immersion in a solution of this substance, not only can the putrefaction of excrement be prevented, but also the evolution from it of the gases and vapours which are injurious to health.

Use of Antiseptics.

The use of antiseptics of various kinds, having the property of preventing the decomposition of organic matters, has been known for ages, and occasionally practised more or less in all times for special purposes. It is, however, only within the last few years that antiseptics, possessing also deodorising

* The substance which forms the active principle in McDougall's disinfecting powder and liquid.

properties, have been brought into notice; particularly those which, under certain circumstances, were not likely to do so much harm in some shape or other as would more than counterbalance their influence as disinfectants, and those which could be obtained at a cost that would not preclude the possibility of their general application.

Dr. Angus Smith, of Manchester, who has made the disinfection of sewage and such matters a particular study for several years, and who is, doubtless, a high authority on such subjects, stated, before the Commissioners appointed to inquire into the Sanitary Condition of the Army in India, that "whenever organic matter begins to decompose, the parts of which it is composed are separated and come out in forms which are hurtful to health; but we can prevent this decomposition from going forward, and we can prevent the formation of those gases or vapours which are hurtful to health." He also gave several beautiful examples of the action of carbolic acid in this process*; which, on account of its combined antiseptic and deodorising properties, and the absence in it of any "striking effect on pure substances, beyond preserving them from decay," he considered to be the best known substance for disinfecting sewage and other decomposing organic matters. The carbolic acid of commerce is made from coal-tar, obtained in the manufacture of gas, by a process which originated with Dr. Angus Smith; and to him

* Minute of evidence by Dr. Angus Smith, F.R.S., Professional Chemist, taken before the Commissioners appointed to inquire into the Sanitary State of the Army in India.—Commissioners' Report, vol. I., p. 155 to 164.

also is due the credit of its introduction as a disinfectant; but for its introduction commercially the public is indebted to the energy of Mr. Alexander McDougall, of Manchester, who brought it out under the name of "McDougall's Disinfecting Powder and Liquid," which he describes as "a compound of two acids and two bases. The acids are sulphurous acid and carbolic acid, and the bases magnesia and lime. These four exist in it as two salts, viz., sulphite of magnesia and lime, and carbolate of lime."

The disinfecting powder is very highly spoken of by the officers in charge of public institutions, where it is in constant use, as a most effectual disinfectant and deodoriser. I have seen it applied in a variety of ways; and its influence in the complete and rapid destruction of the most offensive emanations was always most striking, and all that could be desired. Not the least interesting of such matters is Mr. McDougall's farm at Carlisle, where a hundred acres of grass-land are irrigated with sewage, without the least disagreeable smell being perceptible in any part of the fields. When I visited the place, there was not the slightest offensive effluvium, even about the well where the pump was at work forcing up the sewage. In fact, there was every evidence to show that, immediately the disinfecting substance came into contact with the sewage, all offensive smell ceased,* and the deodorisation was rendered so com-

* In speaking of the effects of the disinfecting substance on sewage, Dr. Smith says:—"When the liquid runs into the sewer the smell ceases, and one may enter without fear or disgust. The sewer-water ceases to putrify; but, lest our judgment on this point may appear somewhat biased, we prefer bringing

plete that, although the sewage was conducted all over the farm in open iron drains, the air was as fresh and pleasant as any meadow in England. The cattle and sheep which were grazing on the sewage pasture appeared in excellent health and condition—one of the best signs of the efficiency of the principle. I was informed that sheep suffering from rot (a parasitic disease already alluded to) were cured by feeding on this kind of pasture. I cannot, however, speak on this point from personal observation; but, if the information be correct, it would be another proof of the value of disinfected sewage as a manure.

I have visited some large stables where carbolate of lime is regularly used as a disinfectant; and not only was the interior of the stables perfectly sweet, but the middens belonging to them, which generally emit most disgusting smells, were perfectly free from all offensive effluvium. I have had the disinfecting powder applied to decomposing farm-manure under my own observation, and have seen its action on recent ordure of all kinds, before and after decomposition had set in, with the same excellent results. I feel perfectly confident that it would supply the great desideratum in Indian conservancy, and that

---

forward the opinions of gentlemen who are quite disinterested. Dr. Bernays, of St. Thomas's Hospital, gave his opinion in the *Lancet*, August 13th, 1859. He found that sewage that was treated in this way remained free from sewage smell even in July; and sewage deposit, which is the worst part of sewage, remains to this day equally beneficially affected. About the same time, Dr. Letheby was requested to give his unbiased opinion; and he undertook experiments, the result of which he has kindly transmitted. They will be found very striking, and completely agree with our long experience, leaving nothing further to desire as to the capacity of the liquid to prevent putrefaction."—"On the Means of Disinfecting Sewage," by Dr. Angus Smith.

its ample and easy applicability adapts it peculiarly for this purpose. As we thus have a substance which puts an immediate stop to the decomposition of sewage, in whatever state of advancement it may be, and destroys in a moment the loathsome effluvium, indescribable in words, that arises from it; and as the substance prevents the decomposition of organic matters from even commencing, we simply want a convenient mode of applying it to newly-voided excrementitious matters, to render it peculiarly useful in the conservancy of public latrines—a matter which can be easily managed by a very simple arrangement.

Latrines.

The latrines for public purposes, manufactured by Messrs. Macfarlane and Co., of the Saracen Foundry, Glasgow, and supplied by them to many of the barracks in England, and, I believe, also to some of the British barracks in the Mediterranean and America, and highly recommended by the commissioners appointed for the improvement of barracks and hospitals, simply require the addition of a reservoir for the disinfecting substance, with suitable apparatus, adjusted for the admission of it into the latrines in a given quantity. This apparatus has been suggested by me, and is shown in Fig. 22 (page 109). It is simple, easily adjusted, and cannot fail in fulfilling the purpose for which it is intended.

In addition to the apparatus for supplying the disinfectant, I have proposed a modification of Macfarlane's latrine, shown in section in Fig. 23 (page 111). This adapts it, by a very simple arrangement, for the double purpose of water-closet and urinal, so that the urine and whole excrementitious matters may be deodorised and disposed of together. I am aware that some objections are likely to be raised to such an arrangement, but the arguments I have heard urged against the principle are not conclusive. Moreover, the different kinds of night-soil are more likely to be thoroughly disinfected and properly disposed of in every way, by the whole process being conducted at the same time and place; and, as there is quite as great reason, perhaps greater, for turning sewage to account as manure in India as in any part of the world, provided the process does not interfere with sanitary conditions; and as urine contains the richest fertilising matter in digested substances, but acts more permanently and beneficially when applied to the soil in combination with the other parts of night-soil, the latrines which embrace the double purpose of water-closet and urinal, will, I feel certain, be found a decided improvement.

The latrines (Fig. 22) consist of an oblong trough, A, in three compartments, the bottom being egg-shaped, with an inclination towards the discharge-end. The discharge-apparatus compartment is separated from the rest of the trough by the sluice-plate, B, sufficient space being left between its under edge and the bottom of the trough to allow the matters to pass freely through to the discharge-pipe. In the bottom of this compartment is the discharge-pipe, C, with socket-valve and overflow waste-pipe, D. These, *i.e.*, the socket-valve and overflow waste-pipe, are in one piece, and connected to the upright link, E,

FIG. 22.

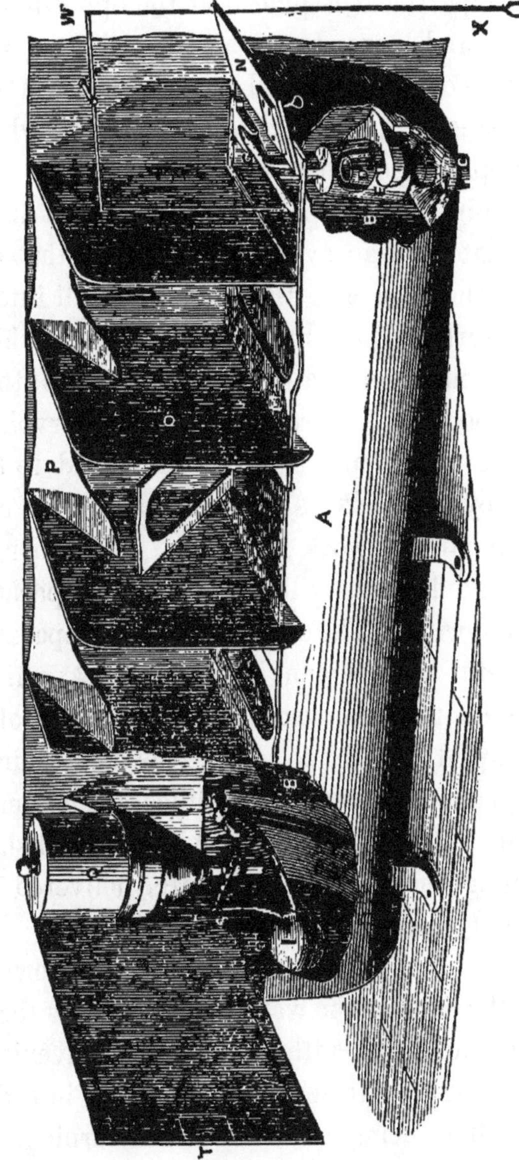

Latrine.—A. Oblong trough. B B. Sluice-plates. C. Discharge-pipe. D. Overflow waste-pipe. E. Upright link, to which the socket-valve and waste-pipe are connected. G. Horizontal lever. I. Float-ball and cock. M. Seat. N. Hinged cover and lock. O. Partition between seats. P. Back-piece for preventing persons from standing on the seat. Q. Deodoriser reservoir. R. Stop-cock and lever. S. Link connecting R to I. T. Door. W. Lever. X. Rope.

which again is acted on and wrought by the horizontal lever, G, the whole being enclosed by the hinged cover and lock, N. The water-supply and deodorising substance compartment is placed at the opposite end of the trough, and consists of a sluice-plate, B, and float-ball and cock, I, attached to the back of the trough by means of a thimble, to the latter of which the water-supply pipe must be soldered. The deodoriser-reservoir, Q, is suspended by a bracket fixed to the back plate or wall over the trough, so that the deodorising substance and the water will fall into it together, as nearly as possible at the same spot, which will facilitate their intimate intermixture as they pass into the body of the trough. The reservoir is fitted with a stop-cock and lever, R, connected to the float-ball, I, by the link, S, so that the water and deodorising apparatus work in unison. The door, T, when closed and locked, will prevent the apparatus being tampered with. The only part of this apparatus requiring careful arrangement is the stop-cock, which, whether the disinfectant used be in the form of a powder or a liquid, must be so adjusted as just to admit the proper quantity required to disinfect the contents of the trough. However, this is easily accomplished by ascertaining the quantity of water delivered by the water-supply-cock in a given time.

Fig. 23 is a cross-section of the latrines, showing the urinal at the back of the water-closet. At U there is a plate 6 inches in breadth, placed at a convenient angle for catching the urine and directing it into the trough; and, there being no complicated turnings in the passage, the whole will be very easily kept clean by hand-scrubbing with a cloth and strong solution of the disinfectant, which should always be used for cleaning these places.

Physiologists generally estimate the quantity of fæces passed by an adult from 5 to 6 ounces, and of urine from 30 to 40 ounces daily, the latter being considerably affected by temperature and other causes; so that, if the average of the two together be put down

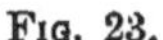

Fig. 23.

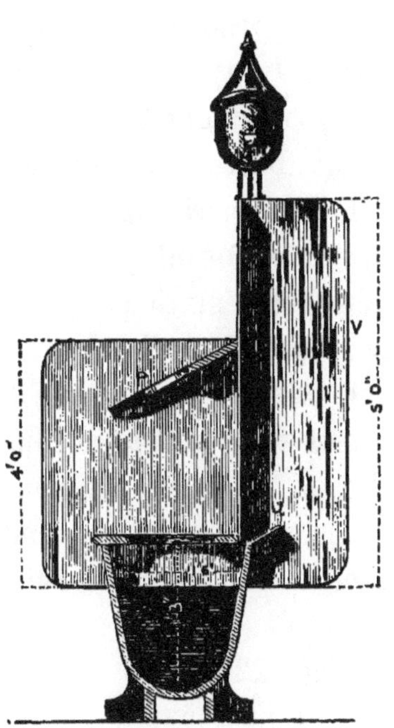

Section of Latrine.—P. Back-piece for preventing persons from standing on the seat. U. Plate for directing urine into trough. V. Wall of urinal.

at 40 ounces for the warm climate of India, which is equal to 4,000 ounces per 100 men *per diem*, the quantity will not be under-estimated.

The proportion of disinfecting powder required for the treatment of a given quantity of night-soil, including urine, has not been determined very accurately. The article being very cheap, the plan pursued hitherto seems to have been to apply plenty of it, so as to insure complete deodorisation; but Dr. Angus Smith states, in relating some of his experiments, "that, with the average quantity of sewage, about 1 per cent. of carbolic acid solution was sufficient to arrest putrefaction, and that with the worst kind of stagnant sewage about 15 per cent. was sufficient;" and, judging from some experiments of my own, and from what I have seen elsewhere of this disinfectant, I believe that about 3 per cent. of the powder would be sufficient to prevent putrefaction of newly voided night-soil, if properly applied, but say 15lbs. per 100 men *per diem* for all purposes, which would perhaps cost about the sixth or seventh of a penny per man at any station in India.

In providing latrines for troops, it is considered that the number of seats should not be under five to every hundred men, exclusive of non-commissioned officers and women.* However, for India the number should be two or three above this ratio, when at all admissible.

A glance at Figs. 22 and 23 will show that, if the latrines are placed in the middle of a moderate-sized apartment, the air will have free circulation round every part of them, as well as every facility and convenience afforded by such a position for keeping the whole place clean; and at the same time

* Report of the Commissioners for Improving the Sanitary Condition of Barracks and Hospitals, page 90.

each compartment would be quite as private as if the latrines were placed against a wall.

In preparing a building for latrines on this principle, it will be necessary to construct a few feet of an arch under the floor, at one end of the apartments, so as to provide a space below it for the ordure-cart (Fig. 24, p. 114) being backed under the discharge-hole, c, of the latrines (Fig. 22). On this arch the discharge-end of the latrines must rest, and the pipe, c, lead through it to the ordure-cart underneath. The part of the floor on which the latrines stand should be covered with large plates of iron or slabs of slate, or other stone, closely jointed together, and so arranged that they could be removed occasionally; and a few inches of the materials underneath them should be renewed if found offensive. The apartment should be provided with ridge-openings for ventilation, and the interior ventilated on the same principle as recommended for the barracks. It should also be well lighted both by day and night. For night purposes, a sufficient number of lamps should be arranged, as represented in Fig. 23, so as to throw a good light over the whole apartment.

The ordure-cart (Fig. 24, p. 114), which must be of a size to hold the whole contents of one trough, consists of a water-tight body or tank, with a small trap-door in the top for receiving the night-soil, and a discharge-valve behind, worked by a long lever, for discharging the contents of the cart at a manure depot, or spreading it over a station farm, as may be desired. If there is not sufficient height between the surface of the ground and the top of the arch mentioned in the last paragraph, to admit the cart under the discharge-pipe of the latrines, an inclined plane, of easy gradient, must be constructed for the purpose; but a much better plan would be to raise the floor of

Fig. 24.

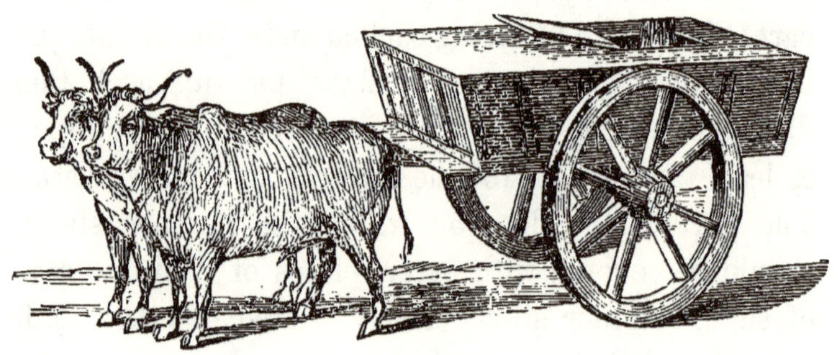

Ordure-Cart.

the latrines sufficiently high above the ground to obviate the necessity of such a roadway. The small trap-door of the cart being brought directly under the discharge-pipe of the latrines, and the rope, x, being pulled, the levers, w and G, are set in motion. This opens the socket-valve, and the whole contents of the latrines are at once discharged into the cart, and the trough is refilled by the self-acting apparatus at the opposite end, already described. The number of carts that will be required for a regiment will depend on the distance the night-soil will have to be carried; but I conceive four, at least, will be necessary—namely, two for the barrack-latrines, including those for the married quarters, one for the hospital, which should be kept for it exclusively, and one for the cook-house. As much of the efficiency of the whole system will depend on this part of the arrangements, these carts should be of the best construction and capacious ; and every care should be taken to keep them in proper working order.

Disposal of Sewage.

For the final disposal of the sewage, station farms should be established of, say, about a hundred acres each to begin with, laid out in grass, on which the whole sewage should be spread by the ordure-carts direct from the latrines. Good grass is always valuable and in demand, particularly at large stations; and the profits of the farm, if properly managed, would very soon be a source of revenue to the conservancy establishment;* or, if the Government should not wish to continue working the farm, after a time natives would very soon be found to take it up ; but the example must be shown by Government in the first instance.

It has already been shown that disinfected sewage may be used as manure without the least inconvenience or bad results ; and, when it is largely diluted with water, it is found that the disinfecting properties of the soil are quite sufficient to prevent any disagreeable consequences, and, in fact, that the best, most beneficial, and profitable way of disposing of sewage, is the direct application of it in the liquid form to land.†

---

* Many instances might be cited of the profits realised from grass lands irrigated with sewage, averaging from a few shillings to £30 and £40 per acre. As an example of the latter, I may mention the Craigentinny Meadows, near Edinburgh, some portion of which has been irrigated with sewage for upwards of sixty years.

† "The most beneficial and most profitable method of disposing of sewage, where circumstances will admit of the use of it, is by direct application in the

With regard to the use of grass grown on sewaged land, I may mention, with the view of removing any prejudices which may exist against it, that the flavour even of the milk of cows fed on it is not in the least affected, and "analysis shows very little difference in the quality of the milk yielded respectively from sewaged and unsewaged grass. The difference in composition, such as it is, is slightly in favour of the milk from the unsewaged grass when grass was given alone, and slightly in favour of the sewaged grass when oil-cake was given in addition."*

Moveable Urinal.

Fig. 25 represents a moveable urinal, to be made entirely of iron, for night purposes, or any other where such articles may be deemed necessary. The discharge-pipe, C, is in the middle of the trough, and consists of exactly the same kind of apparatus as that used for discharging the contents of the latrines: it is secured from being tampered with by the door, H, the key of which should be kept by the person in charge of the conservancy. The urinal consists of a trough, D, 3 ft. square by 1ft. 3in. deep, and four compartments formed by partition-plates, E E, back-plates, F F, and projecting-plates, G,

---

liquid form to land; where such application can only be conveniently effected near habitations, it may be desirable to employ some deodorising agent, but usually, if proper arrangements are made for conveying sewage on to the land, this expense need not be incurred."—Second Report of the Commissioners appointed to inquire into the best mode of distributing the Sewage of Towns, p. 40.

* Second Report of the Commissioners appointed to inquire into the best mode of Distributing the Sewage of Towns, p. 37.

for catching the urine and directing it into the tank.

Fig. 25.

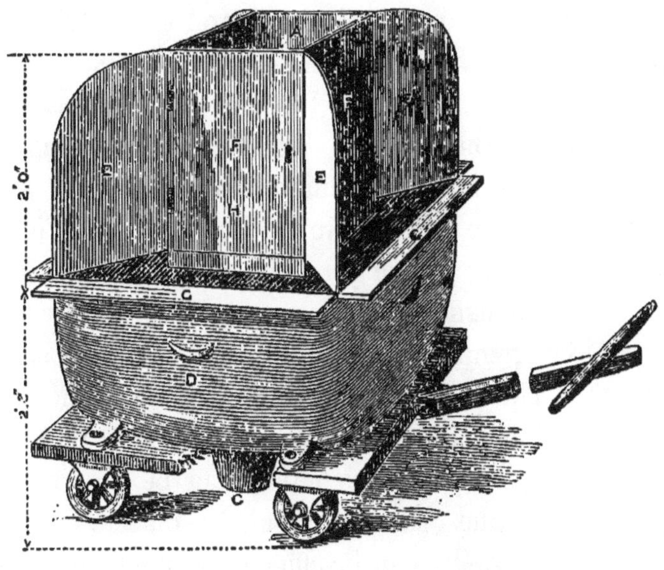

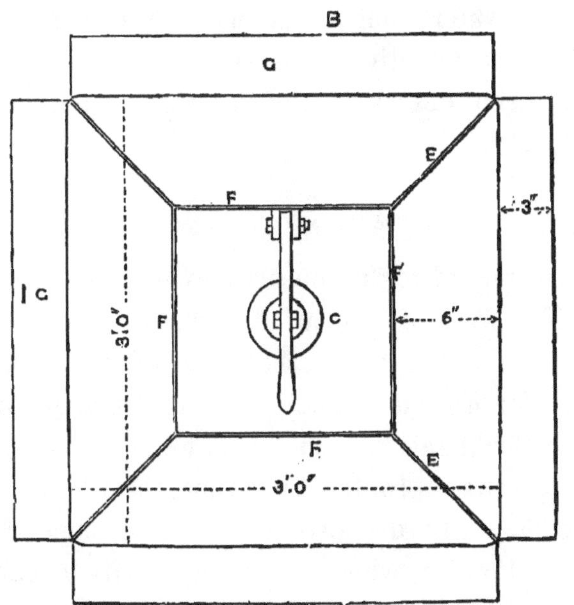

Moveable urinal for four persons.—A. Elevation. B. Transverse section. C. Discharge-pipe. D. Trough. E E. Partition-plates. F F. Back-plates. G G. Projecting-plates. H. Door.

The plates which form the back of each compartment should extend an inch or two into the water. The urinal should be mounted on an iron truck, with the wheels, nine inches in diameter, entirely underneath the platform, which should be a little less in area than the mouth of the trough. The top, which forms the compartments, must be secured to the trough by slip-keys, so as to be easily removed for the purpose of all the parts being thoroughly cleaned. The truck is drawn in the usual way, by a pole and yoke, which should be removed when the urinal is in position for use. The urinals are emptied in the same way as the latrines; and for this purpose a small platform will be necessary on which they can be drawn, and under which the ordure-cart can be placed.

No conservancy can be efficient without a plentiful supply of water; but, as the mode of obtaining it in any required quantity within reasonable bounds has already been described, the description need not be repeated.

Conservancy of Prisons.

With regard to the conservancy of Indian prisons, a modified form of Macfarlane's water-closets, which would not cost one-half the price of those recommended for European soldiers' barracks, might be introduced for the accommodation of natives with equally useful results. In the meantime, the whole of the ordure should be deodorised with McDougall's Disinfecting Powder, which could very easily be effected in the same manner in which open places are disinfected in this country; namely, by sprinkling the places to be disinfected as often as may be necessary with the powder from a common large tin dredger. The latrines should be well sprinkled with the powder at least twice a day; and the water used in cleaning them should be a solution of the powder of a given strength, and for this purpose a small reservoir, containing disinfecting water, should be attached to each latrine. Properly-constructed ordure-carts should be used, and the sewage applied to land belonging to the prison, or sold to any one willing to purchase it for a similar purpose. If the ordure were properly deodorised, it could be removed in the way already recommended at any time, without causing the least nuisance or inconvenience to any one, and would very soon be a source of profit to the prison department, instead of a heavy expense as at present.

Ablution.

With regard to ablution rooms and baths, they should be so placed that the water from them can be used for the irrigation of the gardens. Shower-baths on an economical principle could very easily be arranged in any number, and would be of immense use in a sanitary point of view; and, if they were conveniently situated, I believe the men would use them extensively.

For ablution of all kinds, the apparatus manufactured for the purpose by Messrs. Macfarlane and Co., of Glasgow, is admirably adapted, and should be brought into use as much as possible. The apparatus consists of either a single basin, or single or double ranges of them, each range containing as many basins as may be desired. When in ranges, "each basin occupies a space 1ft. 6in. by 2ft. A bib-cock supplies each basin with water, and a moveable stopper discharges the waste water ; the whole stands on brackets, against the wall or in the middle of the floor, as may be found most convenient. For washing the feet, fixed basins, similar in construction to the wash-hand basins, are also made by Messrs. Macfarlane and Co. Each basin occupies 1ft. 6in. by 2ft., and is 1ft. 2in. from the ground."* The apparatus would answer admirably for India, if the ablution rooms were properly supplied with water.

---

* Report by the Commissioners for Improving the Sanitary Condition of Barracks and Hospitals, p. 99.

CHAPTER VI.

DRAINAGE.

However complete all other sanitary conditions of a locality may be, if not properly drained it cannot be considered healthy; and periodical visitations of disease, assuming epidemic forms, will make their appearance when least expected, in spite of the best conservancy. One of the first sanitary considerations should, therefore, be attention to the drainage, not only on the surface, but to some considerable depth in the subsoil. The natural drainage may be good, and the surface dry; yet the subsoil may be very wet, almost to the surface.*

We frequently hear it remarked, without sufficient reason, that certain stations cannot be drained. There are very few stations that could not be drained; I

---

* On one occasion I selected a site for a large prison, in an open elevated situation; the surface-drainage was good, and the locality apparently well adapted in every way for the purpose, and considered so by the local officers well acquainted with the place. The water in a well in the middle of the site, and in others round about it, was 12 to 15 feet from the surface. In short, the site was altogether a very good one; and during the first rainy season after it was selected, nothing unusual took place to alter the opinion originally formed of it; the water rose a little in the well, but not more than might be expected, and the officer ordered to examine the site from time to time during and subsequently to the rains, sent in a favourable report. However, fortunately the building happened to be delayed for nearly two years, and, in the meantime, the site became almost a swamp; at least, the water rose so close to the surface that it began to ooze up in trenches two and three feet in depth, and rose in the well until it was within three feet of the brink. This, it is true, was during the rainy season, but the same state of things continued for months. The site was, of course, abandoned.

never saw one ; drainage is simply a matter of expense, more or less difficult under certain circumstances, of course, but probably always possible. Stations that cannot be thoroughly drained, if any exist, should be at once abandoned.

In laying down a system of drains for a station, careful arrangements should be made for preventing filth of every kind from being washed into them ; they should not communicate with the interior of any dwelling-house, and the openings should be at a distance from all inhabited places. If, however, they are properly constructed, and nothing but surface and waste water be allowed to run into them, they will very easily be kept clean. Occasional flushing with plenty of water, which the system already described can supply, and a few pounds of the disinfecting powder thrown into them at the conclusion of each flushing, will remove all danger of any disagreeable emanations from them. But to make sure that no foul air is being generated, the air in the drains should be carefully tested at least once a week, and its condition recorded ; and, if it be found in an unsatisfactory state, the drains should be at once flushed and carefully disinfected, until all signs of foul air disappear. In the event of any unusual amount of foul air forming in them, a strong current of air, loaded with the fumes of carbolic acid, should be sent through them by a moveable powerful blower and apparatus for the purpose ; but with good general arrangements this should rarely be necessary. However too great care cannot be observed in preventing the formation of foul air outside as well as inside buildings.

CHAPTER VII.

SUPERVISION.

The various arrangements which compose a regular system of sanitation cannot continue in a state of efficiency without proper supervision, any more than other matters of business or trade which affect the well-being of mankind, and which are supervised with most anxious care ; yet it would seem as if the matters which more directly affect our very existence should in many instances be left to take care of themselves. Even in the simplest form of ventilation, where the apparatus is merely the ordinary doors, windows, and fire-places, constant attention is necessary. If, for instance, the windows of an apartment are never opened, which is too frequently the case, simply through its being no one's business to see that they are so at the proper time, the inmates become poisoned by the exhalations from their own bodies, because the bugbear draught stands ever before them, preventing the admission of fresh air. There is nothing that requires more constant watching than ventilation and conservancy, particularly the former, for the reason that foul and fresh air are equally invisible, and that the evils arising from bad machinery or want of attention to it in this particular matter may proceed to a most dangerous extent, without any of our ordinary senses being cognisant of anything being wrong. Therefore, one of the first points in sanitary arrangements should be the appointment of supervisors, who thoroughly understand sanitary science in all its bearings, with sufficient means at their disposal to enable them to carry out at once such measures as they may deem necessary, and to keep the whole machinery which they may establish in proper working order.

At the places where sanitation is most required, it fortunately so happens that there need be no want of good overseers and first-rate workmen. Wherever there are European soldiers, it would not only be an advantage to the state, but a positive boon to the men themselves, independently of the remuneration which they might receive, to give them healthful employment. With the exception of the principal machinery, such as steam-engines, fans, pumps, and latrines, the greater portion of the work suggested in the foregoing pages might be executed by the soldiers themselves.

In former times, soldiers were not less brave, or fought and conquered with less success, or bore the fatigues of campaigns with less endurance, because they made roads and executed other military work when not required for actual fighting in the field. In storming forts, do men grapple with the foe in the breach with less prowess, because they have worked their way to it through months of hard labour in the trenches and other severe toil? Would a prize-fighter, who had undergone no more severe training than throwing himself into certain attitudes of defence, or a pedestrian who simply exercised his limbs in a quiet morning walk, ever win the prize? Can there be a more apt remark than the common saying that a man, when he appears strong and in robust health, looks like a navvie? But it is not necessary to go to these extremes, to prove that the man who spends his life in idleness and inaction is not the man who is most healthy and who will bear the most fatigue; for we see in every-day life that daily, well-regulated, steady labour keeps men healthy, and renders them strong and robust in every respect; and there can be no doubt that a certain portion of the day passed in steady useful labour would do soldiers an immense deal of good, both in body and mind; and, if sufficient encouragement were given to them, a very large amount of excellent work of all kinds might be turned out by soldiers, many of whom are already first-class workmen. At all events, there would be no difficulty in getting men from amongst them to superintend and work the steam-engines, ventilating apparatus, ice-making machines, and water-works, and to supervise the conservancy arrangements in all their details; and all necessary repairs for machinery, carts, bedsteads, &c., could be executed in the barrack-workshops, so that there would be no difficulty in keeping the whole machinery of the system in working order. Good and sufficient supervision at almost any cost, judiciously laid out, is economy in the end. The scheme which cannot afford it would better be left alone, for without it certain failure must be the result.

There should be inspectors of divisions to

thoroughly supervise the whole scheme, and see it properly worked on true sanitary principles; and, subordinate to them, deputy-inspectors should be attached to certain stations or localities with a staff of overseers, say one to each department, with a sufficient number of workmen for carrying on the details of the work, a certain number of whom, though belonging to the ranks of the army, should not be moved with their regiments, but left for certain periods in charge of the machinery. The whole should be under the inspector of the division, who should have the power to sanction the expenditure of a certain sum periodically, on the usual conditions, so as to enable him to make at once such additions, alterations, and repairs, as he might think necessary, which is the only sure way of securing efficiency.

CHAPTER VIII.

CONSTRUCTION OF BARRACKS.

With regard to the construction of barracks, whether double-storied or not, the ground floor should be well raised, say four feet above the level of the ground; and it should be borne in mind that the cubic contents of an apartment do not always indicate that the inmates have a sufficient supply of pure air, particularly in a hot climate; there must be a certain amount of superficial area as well, otherwise ventilation will be imperfect. Each inmate of an apartment should have at least an area of seventy-two superficial feet, and the beds should be at least four feet apart. The height of an apartment should not be under seventeen feet, and there is very little use in its being more than twenty-four. With sufficient superficial area, seventeen to twenty feet will be quite sufficient; and without sufficient area no amount of air piled above a person's head will render his position either comfortable or healthy. The important fact should never be lost sight of, that no person can live without a certain amount of fresh air, and that in a hot climate the quantity must be, for reasons already stated, greater and in more rapid motion than in a temperate one; and that, whatever the construction of the barracks may be, if the atmosphere be hot, still, and sultry, and the apartments large, and occupied by what is at present usually considered the full complement of inmates, they never can be healthy if provided with no better ventilation than can be obtained through natural sources.

There can be but one opinion regarding the advantages, in a sanitary point of view, and, I believe, in regard to economy as well, of the location of troops or other large bodies of men in small parties in separate apartments. Some of the new, double-storied, one-company barracks, lately erected in India, are said to have cost upwards of 170,000 rupees each. Now a very excellent, substantial house, containing four or five good rooms, each room affording ample accommodation for four men, could be erected for 8,000 rupees; six such houses would accommodate a company, including non-commissioned officers; and four more similar houses, on a slightly modified plan, for married men, would make a total of ten houses for each company, at say an average cost of 80,000 rupees, being less than one-half the sum which is said to have been expended on the immense piles of buildings alluded to, which will certainly have their turn of unhealthiness like their predecessors. When I speak of a house costing 8,000 rupees, I mean one of a permanent description, built as substantially as the barracks in question. Ordinary houses, called bungalows, constructed of the same kind of materials as the old barracks are built of, could be erected for a sum very much under this amount.

CHAPTER IX.

FINANCIAL RESULTS.

Although the following statement does not profess to give a correct estimate of the various schemes detailed in the foregoing pages, still it will give a fair idea of the probable financial results of improved sanitation on the principle suggested.

Probable Cost of Machinery, Buildings, &c., if erected at Agra, supposed to be in position, ready for work for a full Regiment.*

VENTILATION.

	Rupees.
A Steam-engine, 20-horse power, with boiler complete	8,000
Blowing Apparatus, consisting of two Fans, with 48-inch Impellers	1,500
Engine House, including Room for Ice-making Machines ...	5,000
Building, containing Fan-Room, Refrigerating Room, Fresh-air Shaft, Warming Room, &c., exclusive of Warming Apparatus	10,000
Main Flues, 1,000 yards..	10,000
Barrack-Flues, 800 yards	5,000
Diffusion-Pipes, Perforated Zinc Plates, Gratings, &c., and fittings for the same, say	2,500
	Rs. 42,000

* Agra has been selected simply because it is situated in the interior of the country, about 800 miles from Calcutta, nearly the same distance from Bombay, and about 500 from Lahore, therefore the cost of carriage and other rates may be considered a fair average for stations in the interior.

WATER-WORKS.

	Rupees.
Well	4,000
A Pair of Pumps, to lift 5,000 gallons per hour, with fittings	1,800
Filter	3,000
1,000 yards Cast Iron-pipe, eight inches in diameter	6,000
Distribution-Piping of sizes with fittings	1,000
25 Drinking Fountains	1,250
Fittings	450
	Rs. 17,500

Two Ice-making Machines, medium size	4,000
Fittings	500
	Rs. 4,500

CONSERVANCY.

Ten Latrines, with Urinals attached for six persons, each with Deodorising Apparatus complete, at 350rs. each	3,500
Three ditto, small size, for two persons	500
Houses and Fittings	7,000
Four Ordure-Carts, at 450rs. each	1,800
20 Moveable Urinals, with Trucks complete, 125rs. each	2,500
	Rs. 15,300

ABLUTION.

20 Double Ranges of Washhand-Basins, of 8 Basins each, at 200rs. per Range	4,000
20 ditto ditto Washfoot ditto	4,000
50 Shower Baths	500
Fittings	500
Swimming Bath	3,000
	Rs. 12,000

SUMMARY.

Ventilation	42,000
Water-works	17,500
Ice-making Machines	4,500
Conservancy	15,300
Ablution	12,000
Total for 1,000 men in Barracks	Rs. 91,300

CAMP.

	Rupees.
Five Ventilating Machines, each consisting of a pair of small fans, with 16-inch impellers and driving gear complete on carriages, at 400rs. each	2,000
1,000 yards Main Canvas Flue, at 5rs. per yard	5,000
Canvas Diffusion-Tubes	11,500
Carriage	1,000
Four Moveable Filters on Carriages complete, at 330rs. each	1,320
Total for 1,000 men in Camp ....Rs.	20,820

GRAND TOTAL.

For 70,000 Men in Barracks	63,91,000
„ 35,000 „ Camp	7,28,700
Rs.	71,19,700

ANNUAL CHARGES TO BE DEDUCTED.

	Rupees.
Cost of 2,100 Recruits to supply death-vacancies, which would be saved by efficient sanitary arrangements, at 1,000rs. per head	21,00,000
Hospital Charges, which would be saved by ditto	19,40,000
Rs.	40,40,000
	2
Saving in two years ....Rs.	80,80,000

The object aimed at in the above statement has been to show that financial considerations need be no bar to the introduction of the scheme suggested. The cost of machinery, &c., has been purposely noted high; and I believe that the whole could be carried into effect for much less than the sum estimated. The machinery and other articles which would be required from England, are entered at about double the manufacturers' prices; and the rates of building, charges for fitting, and so on, will not, I think, be found under the mark; whereas the charges to be deducted as savings to the state on account of sanitary arrangements are, I believe, considerably under it. The deaths are calculated on 70,000 men, at the ratio of 60 per 1000,* and one half only of the product is taken as preventable by proper sanitary arrangements. Again, the hospital charges are one-half the amount which remains of actual expenditure annually (namely, 58,80,000 rs.), after deducting 20,00,000 rs. for sickness assumed to be inevitable.† A glance at the statement will show that there has been no overstraining to bring down the estimate to the lowest possible figure. Yet, allowing over eight lacs of rupees (8,60,000) for management and working establishment—a sum far beyond what would be necessary—the saving to the state would cover the expenditure in two years, independently of the improved condition of the army and other considerations of equally great importance.

In carrying out such a scheme as has been proposed in the foregoing pages, the most economical, expeditious, and satisfactory plan in every way would be, to have the whole of the machinery and everything required for the purpose, with the exception of such articles as could be made by the soldiers themselves in the barrack-workshops, direct from England. Every article should be selected from the best makers, by a competent person, who would be held responsible that every piece of machinery, &c., was of the best quality and in proper working order before leaving the maker's hands.

---

* Report of the Commissioners appointed to inquire into the Sanitary State of the Army in India, p. 11.

† Report of the Commissioners appointed to inquire into the Sanitary State of the Army in India, p. 18.

It has been suggested that the disinfecting powder should be made in India. This, I think, would be a mistake ; the substance is of too great consequence for the manufacture of it to be entrusted as yet, even in part, to natives; and I fear the process would be left very much in their hands, however much appearances might be to the contrary.

CHAPTER X.

DESCRIPTION OF VARIOUS APPARATUS.

As it may not always be convenient to get a Lloyd's or a Schiele's fan, or an Atkinson's carbon filter, the following remarks and diagrams may be of use to those who wish to add to their present comforts a certain supply of fresh air and pure water.

Thermantidote.

Figs. 26 and 27 represent a noiseless thermantidote, the blower of which I have found to far exceed in power anything I have ever met with in the best Indian thermantidote. The outer case, A, with the exception of having two openings for the egress of the air, is much the same as that of an ordinary thermantidote. The impeller, B, consists of a disc of iron or wood, with curved eccentric fans, C C, bolted or otherwise secured to it. A reference to Fig. 27 will show that the fans taper towards the periphery of the impeller, which is keyed to the axle in the usual way. Two thick collars of iron or wood, fitting tightly to the axle, should be bolted to the disc, one on each side, which will have the effect of keeping it steady, and will act on the principle of the collars of a circular saw in making it run fair. The tattie-frame, E, is much larger than generally used;

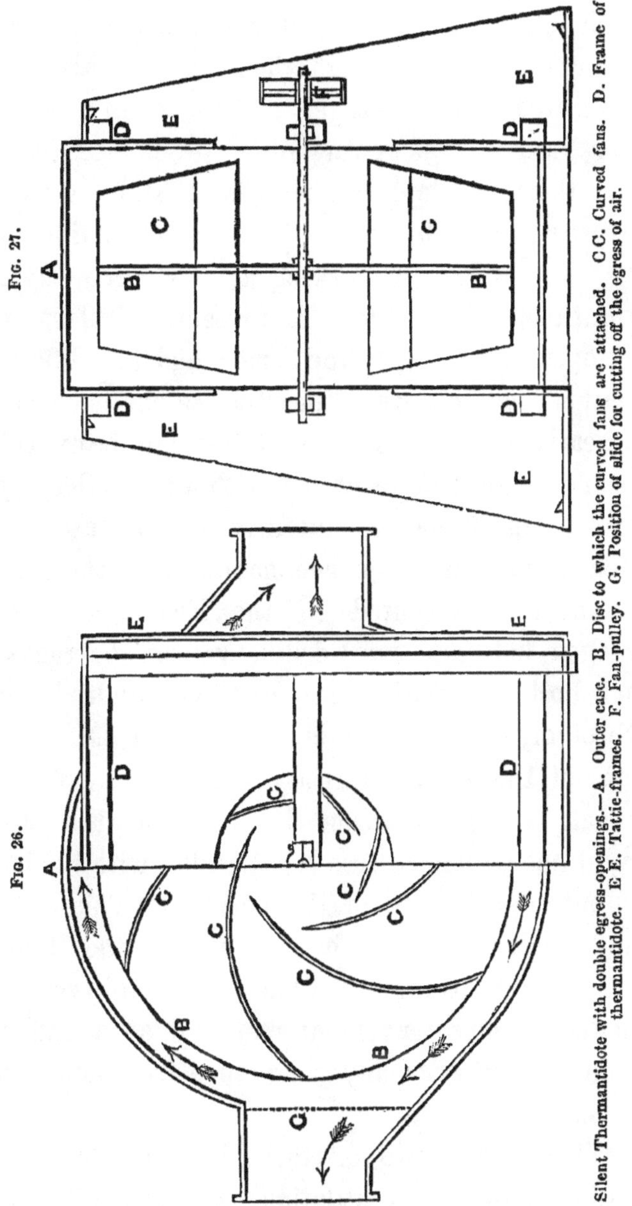

Silent Thermantidote with double egress-openings.—A. Outer case. B. Disc to which the curved fans are attached. C C. Curved fans. D. Frame of thermantidote. E E. Tattie-frames. F. Fan-pulley. G. Position of slide for cutting off the egress of air.

but this is a great advantage, and the relative quality

of thermantidotes very much depends on the size of this useful appendage. When the tatties are small, and the blower is working at even a moderate speed, the air is drawn through them too quickly to be refrigerated in its passage; and the consequence is, that a good blower is very often pronounced useless as a thermantidote. There is a slide at G, for converting the blower into a single-action one. When the blower is working at fair speed, say 250 revolutions per minute, the pressure of blast from each opening is nearly the same; and the difference at either opening, when the opposite one is closed, is not nearly so great as might at first sight be expected. If a blower on this principle, with an impeller, say of four feet in diameter, and driven at a fair speed, which could easily be commanded with the driving machinery represented in the Frontispiece, were arranged between two ordinary-sized barracks or other buildings within two or three hundred feet of each other, it would be quite sufficient to ventilate them on the system already described. When a barrack is ventilated on this principle, the blower should not be placed in a line parallel with the building, but opposite one of the corners. This has the double advantage of being out of the line of natural ventilation, and admits of the blower being situated in any convenient spot, and at a sufficient distance to obviate any annoyance from noise made by those in charge.

Where only two or three buildings are to be ventilated, or the ventilation is required for temporary purposes only, it would be more economical to have the motive power driven by bullocks or horses, than by steam. One good bullock or horse would be quite sufficient to drive a thermantidote such as the one represented above, or a pair of small Lloyd's fans, as represented in the Frontispiece. The machinery is very light, portable, admirably adapted for the purpose, and not expensive. The driving machinery costs, in England, about £13 (130 rs.), and might be set up in almost any part of India for about 250 rupees.

Portable Blower.

Figs. 28 and 29 (p. 138) represent a very convenient kind of portable blower, which could be made up by any handy mechanic for one quarter of the expense, and in less than one half the time, that would be required for making a common thermantidote. A is a common cask of any size,* with the ends removed; B, the fan-frame, which is secured to the cask by four small bolts; C C represents a fan, arranged in some measure on the principle of the Archimedean screw; the leaves, of which there are four, are secured to the axle by the arms D, at about an angle of 35°. If the axle, which should be square except at the bearings, is slightly twisted, say the sixth of a turn, the corners of the bar will take the form of a screw, and the leaves, which should be of thin wood or sheet iron, and about four inches shorter than the cask, when bolted to the arms, will also readily take the screw form.

* The one used in the experiments I conducted in testing the quality of such a blower is an old 35-gallon beer-cask, such as those sent out to India with beer for the troops, and to be had almost anywhere now-a-days for a rupee or so.

The angle of the leaves can be increased or decreased

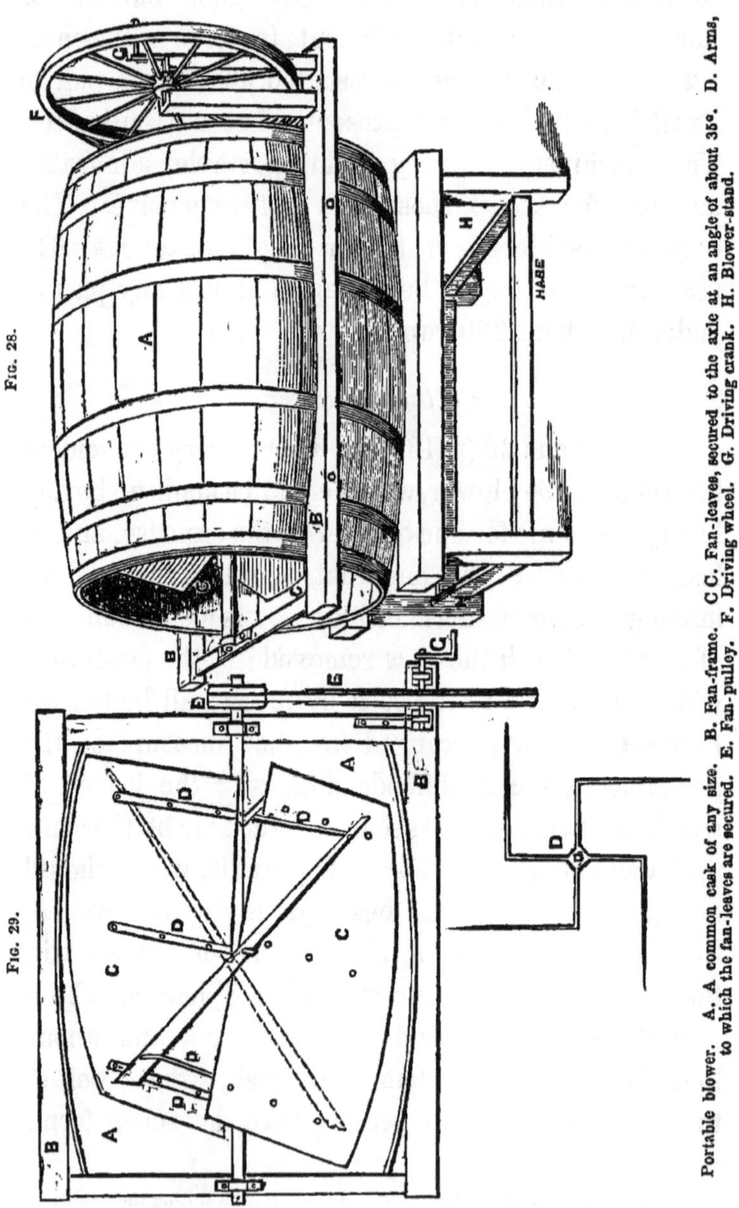

Fig. 28.

Fig. 29.

Portable blower. A. A common cask of any size. B. Fan-frame. C C. Fan-leaves, secured to the axle at an angle of about 35°. D. Arms, to which the fan-leaves are secured. E. Fan-pulley. F. Driving wheel. G. Driving crank. H. Blower-stand.

by simply moving the two outside arms closer to or

farther from the middle one. The fan is driven by a driving wheel, pulley, and belt, in the usual way. The blower may be placed on a wooden stand, H, or arranged in any other convenient mode. A tattie-frame can be adjusted to this blower as easily as to any other. When the cask, which forms the case of the blower, is alone used, the air issues from the mouth of it in what may be called the form of a funnel, and there is almost a calm in the centre of the blast; and when the fan is revolving at great speed there is a very slight reflex current; but these are prevented by attaching a tube of any kind to the discharge-opening of the blower, which may be either another cask, or, what is better and more convenient, a canvas tube of the same diameter as the blower, which may be made of any convenient length, so as to keep the blower well away from the house or tent to which it belongs.

To obviate noise, all machinery employed close to dwelling houses should be worked by frictional gearing and belts, instead of the ordinary toothed wheels.*

Portable Filter.

Figs. 30 and 31 (p. 140) represent a portable filter, which can also be made by any common carpenter or blacksmith. A reference to Fig. 17 (p. 68) will show that the filter is arranged on exactly the same principle as the filter recommended for filtering water on a large scale. A is a common bucket or

* The frictional gearing made by Mr. Robertson, of Glasgow, is almost noiseless, and is admirably suited for ventilating machinery.

other vessel of convenient size; B, a diaphragm placed two or three inches from the bottom of the vessel, so as to allow the water to pass freely under it; C, a partition between the charcoal and sand divisions and the reservoir for filtered water. This partition should be slipped into grooves in the sides and bottom

FIG. 30. FIG. 31.

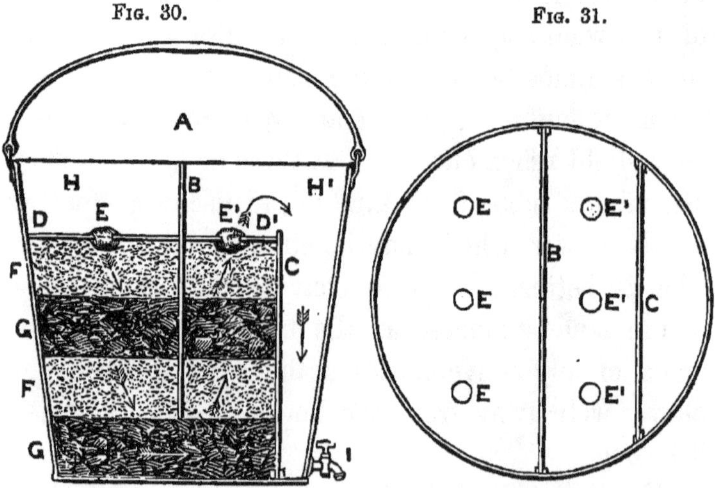

Portable filter. A. Common bucket or other vessel of convenient size. B. Diaphragm of filter. C. Partition between filter and reservoir. D D. Filter cover. E E. Sponge-holes in filter cover. F F. Sand and very small stones. G G. Charcoal. H H. Reservoirs for unfiltered and filtered water. I. Stop-cock.

of the vessel, or into slots, secured to them for the purpose. D D is a cover for keeping the sand and charcoal in position: it should be fitted with small slip-bolts, for preventing them from falling out should the filter at any time be upset; E E are holes in the cover, which, if properly filled up with pieces of sponge, will clear the water from mechanical impurities; F F represents sand and very small stones; G G, charcoal; H H, reservoirs for filtered and unfiltered water; I, a stop-cock. It may not always be convenient to get a stop-cock, but a piece of bent tube can always be procured, and the water drawn off by a siphon in the usual way; and this would perhaps be the better plan of the two, as the siphon would be less likely to get broken or otherwise put out of order. If a wooden vessel be used, the charcoal and sand should be taken out occasionally, and a little burning charcoal put into it for a few minutes, which will destroy any fungi or other vegetable impurities which may form in it or be adhering to the woodwork.

Ambulance.

One or other of the ambulances already in use in Europe are almost as convenient as could be desired; certain modifications, however, would, I think, be an advantage, particularly for India, where such vehicles are most useful on other occasions than the battle-field, and where a great part of the roads are very bad. Crank-axles, of greater length of crank than any hitherto in use for ambulances, so as to admit of the body of the vehicle being hung on its wheels as low as possible, say within a foot or fifteen inches of the ground, would be a great improvement. In this there would be several advantages; and amongst them may be mentioned the reduction of lateral swing, through the body being placed close to the centre of motion, the ease with which the sick or wounded could be placed in them, and the almost impossibility, under ordinary circumstances, of being upset.

Fig. 32 (p. 142) represents an ambulance which was designed by me in 1857, and, with the exception of the crank-axle, is the same as one I sent to Meerut, in the month of March, 1858, for the inspection of Dr. Campbell McKinnon, then Superintendent-Surgeon of that division,* and subsequently forwarded to Allahabad, by desire, for the inspection of the late

Fig. 32.

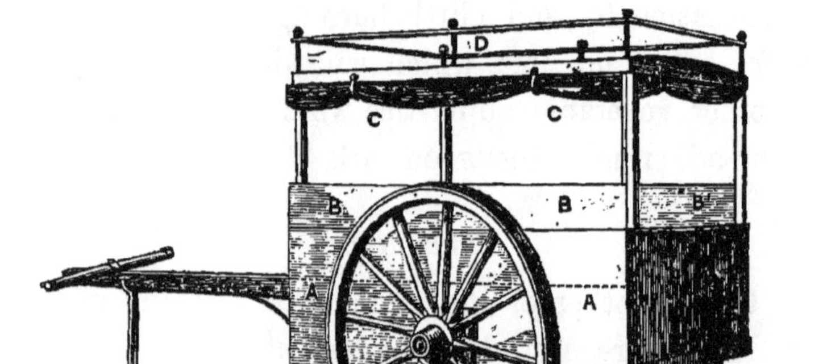

Ambulance.—A. Dotted line showing the position of seat. B B. Wooden flap on hinges, which can be put up or down as required. C. Canvas curtains. D. Iron railings for the protection of baggage.

Lord Canning, then Governor-General of India. The dotted line, A, shows the position of the seat inside; B, a wooden flap, on hinges, which can be shut or open, as may be desirable. C represents canvas curtains rolled up; by the proper adjustment of these two appendages, the occupants of the vehicles

* Dr. C. McKinnon requested me to give him a description of an ambulance suitable for India, which he had heard had been designed by me. This request was complied with; and, at the same time, a vehicle of a temporary kind was forwarded for his inspection, which I begged he would also submit for the opinion of any other person or special committee if he thought proper, and favour me with the result. The only improvement suggested was four wheels instead of two; and, if I remember well, in my subsequent offer to supply any number of such vehicles for the use of the army, it was suggested that a certain proportion, for use on good roads, should be four-wheeled.

can be defended from the chill night-air, from the cutting cold winds which blow during the early mornings in the cold season, and from the glare of the mid-day sun. D is an iron railing for the protection of baggage. The ambulance is fitted with two stretchers, stowed away under the roof when not in use, and is designed for the conveyance of two and even three men in an emergency, lying down with an attendant; or of four reclining with an attendant; or of seven sitting up. In the description which accompanied the ambulance, it was proposed that a number of boxes, of a given size, that could be packed into the ambulances without loss of space or trouble, should always be kept in readiness for medical stores, instruments, and comforts for the sick and wounded; and also that each vehicle should have permanent fixtures for tumblers, bottles, and other necessary vessels, and also racks for arms and such other conveniences as would render the conveyance of sick or wounded men as comfortable as possible.

*Air-Test.**

Although it is now generally known that the presence of organic impurities in air and water can be detected by permanganate of potash, a convenient apparatus for the application of the test has hitherto been a desideratum, which the instrument represented in the accompanying diagrams (33, 34, 35, page 145) is designed to supply. It may not, in its present state, meet all the requirements of the philosophic experi-

* The manufacturer of the Air-Test Apparatus here described is L. P. Casella, 23, Hatton-garden, London.

mentalist; but, in the hands of any one of ordinary intelligence, it will afford an easy and ready means of ascertaining the condition of the air we breathe and the water we drink, as far as the presence of organic matters are concerned, with sufficient precision for all sanitary purposes.

The apparatus consists of a stand, to which a test-tube and moveable scale are adjusted. The scale is composed of a series of ten hermetically sealed tubes, nine of which contain a fluid representing the shades of a solution of permanganate of potash of a given strength, and the tenth is colourless.*

Fig. 33 represents the different parts of the apparatus intact. A is a white porcelain or enamelled plate, 3¼ inches square, with fittings for securing the test-tube, and openings through which the scale is viewed. B is a moveable scale (represented enlarged in Fig. 35), the degrees of which consist of hermetically sealed glass tubes, 2 inches in length by half an inch in diameter, filled with a coloured fluid representing a series of the shades of permanganate of potass, in given quantities, in solution. The first degree, or deepest colour, is equivalent in density to the colour produced by ·0068 grain of the permanganate dissolved in 200 grains of distilled water; and the shades

---

* The idea was taken from a simple contrivance I have long been in the habit of using in the registration of ozone tests. The shades of the ozone scale are painted on a slip of cardboard, and viewed through an opening two inches by three-fourths of an inch, cut in a second piece of card, on which is laid the ozone test to be registered; and the registration is effected in exactly the same way as is laid down for the air-test. The chief advantages in the case of ozone tests consist in cutting off from view all the degrees of colour, except the one under comparison, and the ready means of effecting this object.

of the other degrees of the scale are produced by reducing the quantity of permanganate to the above

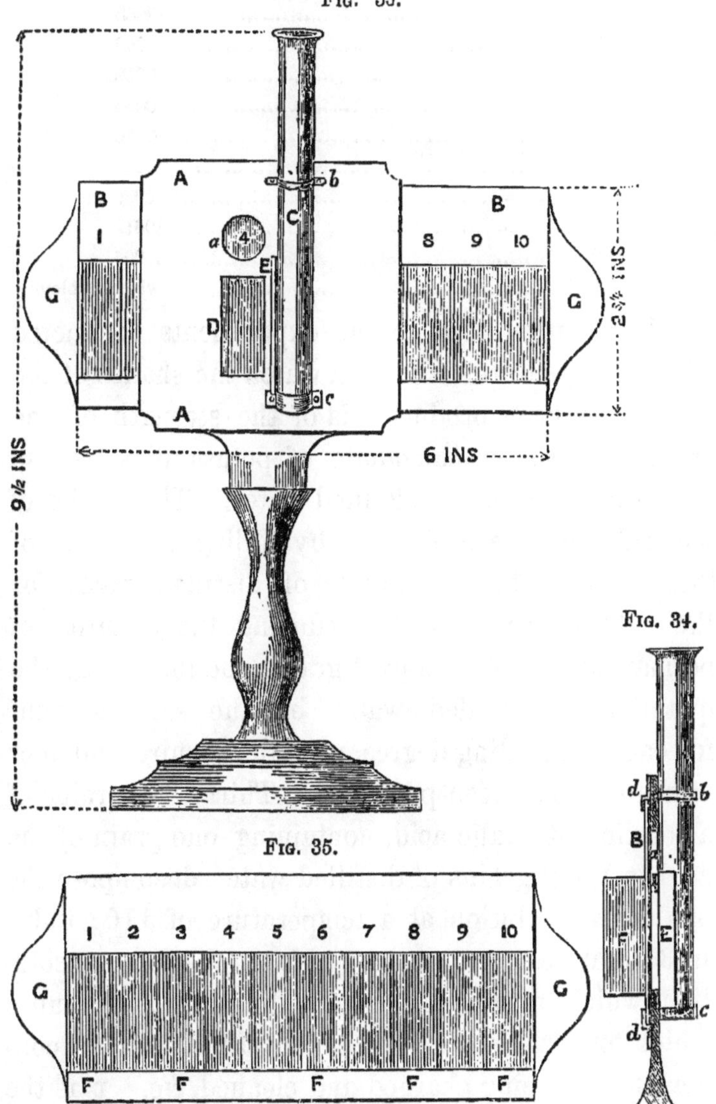

These three figures represent an apparatus for testing air or water. A. Porcelain plate 3¼ inches square. B. Scale-slide. C. Glass test-tube. D. Opening for comparing test with coloured scale. E. Slip for preventing the reflection of colour from the scale to the test, or *vice versa*. F. Divisions of coloured scale. G. Handles of slide. *a*. Registration-hole. *b*. Clamp for securing test-tube to plate. *c*. Shoe of test-tube. *d*. Clamp for slide.

quantity of water, in the following ratio. The tenth degree represents the solution completely decolorised.

	Grain.
1	·0068
2	·0060
3	·0052
4	·0044
5	·0036
6	·0028
7	·0020
8	·0012
9	.0004
10	without colour.

The solution used in the experiments conducted with this apparatus, and from which the shades of the scale have been produced, is of the strength of one grain of pure permanganate of potass dissolved in 2500 grains of newly distilled water. The shades of the scale have been obtained by adding 17 grains of this solution to 183 grains of distilled water for the first degree, and by reducing the quantity of permanganate solution by 2 grains and increasing the quantity of distilled water by the same amount for each succeeding degree, until the required number of shades have been produced. Thirty-five grains of a solution of oxalic acid, containing one grain of the acid to 1,500 grains of distilled water, decompose the one degree solution at a temperature of 110° Fahr. in 35 minutes. C represents a glass tube for test solution, which must be of the same diameter as the tubes which form the scale; it is moveable, for the convenience of being charged and cleaned, &c. D is the opening through which the scale is viewed. E represents a ledge for preventing the reflection of colour from the scale to the test, and *vice versa*.

I have not yet had an opportunity of conducting a sufficient number of experiments with this instrument, with that degree of care which would enable me to state with certainty the amount of organic matter which each degree of the scale indicates. I have, however, made observations with it on the respired air of different individuals, taken at different times of the day and night, and kept for periods ranging from one to twenty-four hours; on the atmosphere of close rooms where several persons were living together; on the emanations from covered house-drains and such places. The quantity of air used in each experiment has been 70 cubic inches, and the test that, of course, given for the first degree of the scale; and I consider that, immediately when the decolorisation falls below the second degree, the atmosphere is sufficiently impure to become unhealthy, and that no time should be lost in improving the ventilation and conservancy of localities where such an indication would be given.

Fig. 36 (p. 148) represents a glass receiver on stand, for the impregnation of air or water with the permanganate test. When the receiver is to be used, it must be filled with distilled or filtered rain-water, and placed in the locality from which the air for observation is to be taken, and the stop-cock at each end opened. As the water runs out at one end of the receiver, the air will rush in at the other; and, as soon as the whole of the water has escaped, both the stop-cocks must be shut, when the receiver may be removed to any convenient place for the completion of the observation, which may be deferred for any length of time. The receiver is mounted on a stand, and fitted with a crank for turning it, which affords easy means of thoroughly impregnating the test with its contents. A receiver of this description would

FIG. 36.

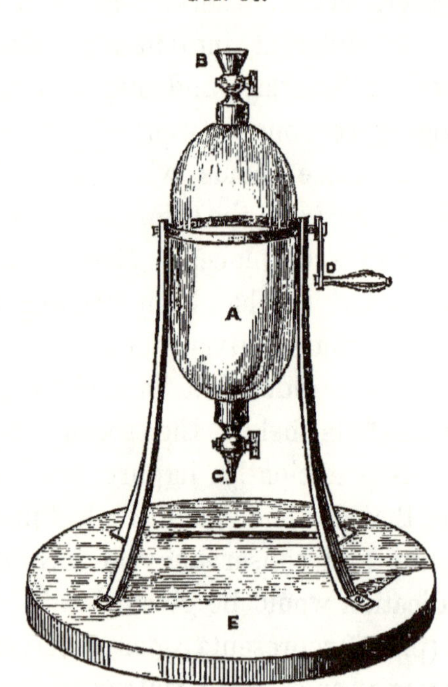

Glass receiver with stand, for impregnating air or water with tests. A. Receiver. B B. Entrance-opening with stop-cock. C. Exit-opening with stop-cock. D. Handle. E. Stand.

be convenient for hospitals, and other places where it might be desirable to have several observations taken during the night-time. Two or more receivers could be prepared and placed under the charge of a night-attendant, who could conduct the first stage of the observations at any fixed periods, and lay by the apparatus until it would be convenient to apply the test.

Fig. 37 represents a more portable receiver, which consists of a bottle of given capacity, having a mouth at each end, and a leathern strap attached, by which it is carried and held in any required position.

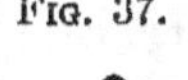

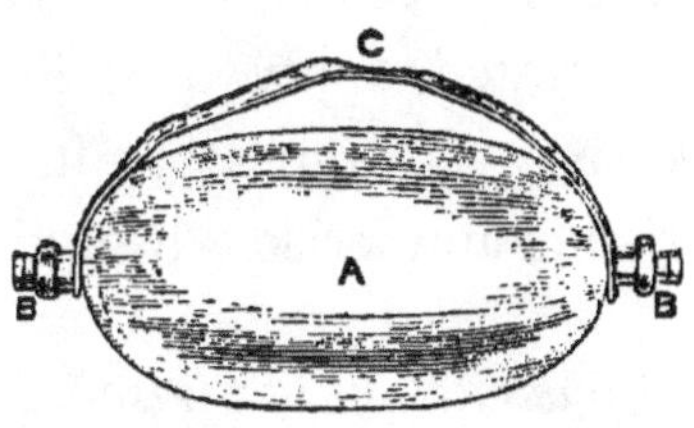

Portable glass receiver for impregnating air or water with tests. A. Glass vessel of any convenient size. B B. Bottle with mouth at each end. C. Leathern strap.

As it is desirable that the observations should be conducted in as simple a form as possible, everything likely to complicate matters should be avoided. If the temperature be low, a longer time will be required for the completion of each observation; but the heat of the hand will be sufficient for all ordinary purposes. The tube containing the test should be held in the palm of the closed hand for a few minutes, so as to communicate a uniform degree of heat to its contents, after which it may be placed in position for comparison with the scale. I find that, when the oxidising solution is maintained at a temperature of 95 to 100 degrees Fahrenheit, the decolorisation gains its minimum in five to six hours; but it would be well to allow longer time when convenient.

As the permanganate solution undergoes oxidation by keeping, it should by prepared immediately prior to being used as an air or water-test; and a portion of the solution employed should be compared with the first degree of the scale, before being submitted for impregnation with the fluid in the receiver.

CHAPTER XI.

PRISONS AND PRISON-DISCIPLINE.

The general principles of ventilation and conservancy of barracks for troops will, with certain modifications already stated, apply to Indian prisons, and therefore need not be repeated in the following remarks on Prisons and Prison-discipline.

Construction of Prisons.

It has already been demonstrated that, wherever large numbers of men are congregated, even in the open air, the atmosphere becomes impure, and outbreaks of epidemics are almost always the consequence; it is therefore most desirable that, whenever it becomes necessary to mass large bodies of human beings together, every means should be adopted for the prevention of this accumulation of impure air, and one of the best is to change the locality of persons so situated as frequently as possible. The benefit derived by sick persons from a removal, even from one room to another, is well understood; and although the benefit of such a slight change would not be so apparent in persons in health, still no one will doubt the great advantage of even slight changes to men confined for long periods within a limited space.

The soldier generally leaves his barrack and its immediate vicinity and breathes the air of some other locality for, at least, a short time every twenty-four hours; and if there is any movement in the atmosphere, a great portion of the impure air which has accumulated in and around his quarters during the night-time is carried off, and he returns to a place which has been well ventilated during his absence. But with the prisoner the case is widely different. He is confined continuously within a certain space, surrounded by high walls; and his greatest change during the twenty-four hours is, at most, a few yards, namely, from his barrack or cell to his workshop or exercising-ground; and within this limited space he eats, sleeps, and labours from one end of the year to the other.

It would be a very simple matter to remedy this state of things without adding materially to the cost of prison-buildings, or abating the necessary amount of prison-discipline. The new prisons in the North West Provinces,* which are admirably adapted for carrying out a regular system of strict discipline, have the workshops in which the prisoners labour within the barrack-enclosures. Each barrack has

* The late Mr. W. Woodcock, of the Bengal Civil Service, first Inspector of Prisons in the North-West Provinces, was the originator of radiating prisons in India; and to him are we indebted for the design of a prison, the general plan of which is admirably suited for hot climates. His successors have altered and modified the plan to meet the increasing wants of the department; it is, however, only simple justice to the memory of this energetic officer, who may be considered the Howard of India, but whose measures have not always received the acknowledgment due to them, to state that the general outline and chief principles of the design remain the same as the plan submitted by him in 1847, and published in 1852 in his final Report on the Prisons of the North-West Provinces.

its suit of workshops, and the men never leave the immediate vicinity of their quarters: this, on sanitary principles, is decidedly objectionable. Now I consider that the workshops should be in separate inclosures, and the system of discipline so arranged as to admit of the daily removal of the prisoners to some little distance from their sleeping quarters, during the hours allotted to labour, which would afford an opportunity for the complete ventilation of the interior of the prison during the day time, and of the workshops at night. The workshops are already separate buildings; so that, in the construction of new prisons, the additional expense would only be the cost of divisional and inclosing walls—an expenditure which would soon be repaid by the reduction in hospital charges and the generally improved condition of the prisoners, who would thereby be enabled to perform a better day's labour. The accompanying ground plan of a central prison for 2,500 prisoners would, I believe, meet the requirements alluded to, as well as admit of the introduction of an improved system of prison-discipline, which would still further improve the sanitary condition of the prisoners.

Prison-Discipline.

It would be impossible to discuss all the phases of prison-discipline in the space which can be allotted here to the subject. Such a discussion, moreover, would be perhaps out of place in a treatise of this kind. I shall, therefore, confine the following remarks chiefly to points bearing more or less on the sanitary condition of the inmates of our Indian prisons.

GROUND PLAN OF A CENTRAL PRISON FOR 2500 PRISONERS

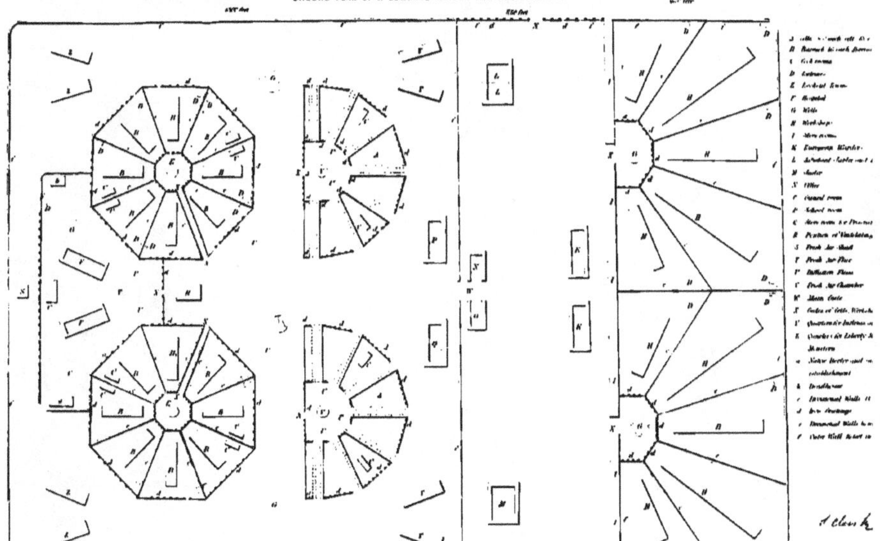

The opinions of men who take an interest in such matters, appear to be almost equally divided regarding the relative advantages of the two systems of prison-discipline in force at present; namely, the system which requires the original sentence to be carried out in full, according to the very letter of the law; and that which contemplates the reformation of the prisoner through a carefully regulated course of prison-discipline resulting in remission of a portion of the original sentence, generally known as the Irish system.

I have always been strongly in favour of giving every prisoner at least one chance of reforming and gaining his livelihood by honest industry, after leaving the prison,* and consider that no system

---

* "Agriculture, as a means of employment for Indian convicts, has not hitherto been attempted, but the marked success which has attended the cultivation of convict farms in other parts of the world is full of encouragement; and I feel confident that a properly managed farm, subordinate to each central prison, would prove of immense advantage in various ways, not the least of which would be affording available ready means of change of air and out-door labour for the weakly prisoners, and enable the superintendent to employ his convalescents profitably, instead of being at a loss, as at present, for something to divert their thoughts from their miserable state, always more or less the reason of slow restoration to perfect health, and not unfrequently the direct cause of relapse.

"The proportion of the convicts in confinement having passed a fixed probationary period in complete incarceration, should also be selected to pass the remainder of their sentence at these farms, under various degrees of surveillance, to be regulated under certain badges and tickets-of-leave.

"Under proper management waste lands might be reclaimed, new systems of agriculture and horticulture brought into play, improved management of live-stock introduced, and, in short, a stimulus given to agriculture in all its phases, a most important branch of industry very much neglected in India, but fully as deserving our best attention as industrial manufactures.

"The chief part of the produce of these farms would be consumed by the prisoners themselves; any surplus, with the exception of live-stock, would be

of prison-discipline can be good which has not this most desirable object in view. This can only be arrived at through careful training in prison, which should, from first to last, tend to make the prisoner feel that the infringement of the laws of the land is no light matter, and at the same time lead him, through judicious relaxation of discipline and a certain amount of indulgence, depending on steady industry and general good conduct, to see that living by honest labour is a much more pleasant way of getting through life than the uncertainty and hardships that attend a system of preying on his fellow-men, or of living in any way in opposition to the laws of his country.

The correctness of these views has been confirmed by my late visits to the prisons and reformatories of this country and of Ireland. I feel quite convinced that the proper way to deal with convicts, so as both to preserve them in health and to prevent their return to their former habits, is to subject them first to a probationary period of severe punishment in confinement. This should be succeeded by intermediate

---

chiefly in cotton, oil-seeds, hemp, and vegetables, which would always find a ready market; in fact, the cotton, hemp, and oil-seeds would be disposed of to the prison manufacturing department at market prices, and a market well supplied with good fresh vegetables would be a real boon to the neighbouring population.

" The present cost of farm and garden produce which is consumed annually at a central prison amounts to upwards of 40,000 rupees. A farm consisting of 1,100 acres in full cultivation at each prison, would supply, in addition to other kinds of produce, the greater part of the cereals required for the use of the prisoners; and the profits on the entire produce, which with few exceptions would be transferred to the prison department at the market rates of the day, would nearly cover the cost of feeding the inmates."—Special Report on the Central Prisons in the North-West Provinces, 1860, by Stewart Clark, Inspector-General of Prisons, N.W.P.

stages of discipline, carried out in the cultivation of prison-farms and other kinds of industrial labour, under the immediate control of the prison authorities. Afterwards, certain indulgences during confinement should be granted to those deserving them; and, finally, a portion of the original sentence should be remitted.

Certain punishments are fixed by law for certain crimes; but, when sentence of a given period of hard labour is awarded to any person for having committed some specified crime, the judge in passing sentence does not contemplate that the convict's health shall be injured in the execution of this sentence, or that his life shall be shortened by the treatment which he may receive during confinement. On the contrary, the intention is that he should leave prison, at the expiration of his sentence, improved in mind, and at least with unimpaired health; therefore every reasonable means should be taken for securing these desirable ends.

In the furtherance of these views, every convict on reception should be placed for five months in strict separate confinement; during which period the punishment should be as deterrent as possible, so as to accustom him to habits of order, cleanliness, and obedience, preparatory to living in association. A remission of one month of the separate confinement should be allowed for good conduct. At the termination of this probationary period, the prisoner should be passed into association in the class assigned to him, and be employed in the workshops on such work as he might be considered fit to perform, for a period consisting of at least three-fifths of the original sentence, under a carefully regulated system of good conduct marks and badges, which, in addition to good conduct, must be determined by the actual amount of work performed or by a decided willingness to work. This term of secondary training should consist of fixed degrees of discipline depending on good conduct, which would entitle the prisoner to certain badges, gratuities, and indulgences; but the full term specified above should be passed strictly within the precincts of the prison. Should the prisoner now exhibit unmistakeable signs of being reformed, and have proved himself deserving of trust and further indulgence, he should be eligible for transfer to the Industrial Department at the convict-farm, and be employed in agriculture, or such other work as he might be best qualified to perform, for a period of at least one-fifth of the original sentence; after which he should receive a ticket-of-leave for employment in any government establishment where his services might be required, under a certain amount of surveillance, or should have a complete remission of the remainder of the original sentence, provided he has proved himself deserving of such great indulgence.*

Under such a system of punishment, carried out in a prison constructed on the accompanying plan, each convict would have an ample supply of fresh air; his mind would be diverted by having some

* My space will not admit of full details, but the system here advocated has been partially carried into effect in the prisons of the North-West Provinces, and the details are given in the Report already quoted and in the prison manual compiled by me in 1862.

certain object to work for; his health would improve instead of deteriorate; and, in all probability, he would leave prison a reformed character, both able and willing to gain his livelihood by honest industry.

A more healthy-looking body of labourers could not be seen, than the prisoners employed on the convict farm at Dartmoor and on the works at Portland, in England, and Spike Island, in Ireland. Those employed at the Smithfield and Lusk Intermediate Prisons in Ireland appear like so many free labourers, with the exception that they carry on their work in a quieter and more orderly manner. In walking over the convict farm at Lusk, the first feeling is astonishment, that a system which appears to work so well should not have been more widely adopted; and the next is, that it must sooner or later become general.

WORKS CONSULTED.

ABEL and BLOXAM. Hand-book of Chemistry.
ARNOTT, J., M.D. Memorandum on Cholera as influenced by Atmospheric Impurity.
BARKER, T. H., M.D. Malaria and Miasmata. Fothergillian Prize Essay.
BERNAYS, A. J., Ph. D. Science of Home Life.
BOWMAN, J. E. Practical Chemistry.
CHRISTISON, R., M.D. Treatise on Poisons.
CONDY, H. B. Air and Water, and their Impurities.
COPLAND, J., M.D., F.R.S. Dictionary of Practical Medicine.
——— Drainage and Sewerage of Large Towns: their Evils and Cure.
GAIRDNER, W. T., M.D. Public Health in relation to Air and Water.
HASSALL, A. H., M.D. Food and its Adulterations.
JEFFREYS, JULIUS. State of the British Army in India.
JOHNSTON, Professor. Agricultural Chemistry and Geology.
——— Analysis of Soils.
KIRKES, W. S., M.D. Hand-book of Physiology.
LANKESTER, E., M.D., F.R.S. Guide to the Food Collection of the South Kensington Museum.
——— Popular Lectures on Food.
LIEBIG, Baron. Chemistry of Agriculture.
——— Familiar Letters on Chemistry.
——— Animal Chemistry.
MACPHERSON, HUGH, M.D. Analysis of later Medical Returns.
MARCET, WILLIAM, M.D. On Food.
MARTIN, Sir J. R., C.B. Influence of Tropical Climates on European Constitutions.
MILLER, W. A., M.D., F.R.S. Elements of Chemistry.
REID, D. B., M.D. Illustrations of Ventilation.
RITCHIE, R. Treatise on Ventilation.
ROBERTSON, W. T., M.D. Sanitary Science: its past and present state.
SNOW, JOHN, M.D. Cholera.
TODD, R. B., M.D., F.R.S., and BOWMAN, W., F.R.S. Physiological Anatomy and Physiology of Man.
TOMLINSON, CHARLES. Warming and Ventilation.
Board of Health Reports.
Journal of the Royal Agricultural Society.
——— Chemical Society.
Popular Science Review.
Report of Commissioners appointed to inquire into the Cholera Epidemic of 1861 in Northern India.
——— of Royal Commission on the Sanitary State of the Army in India.
——— of Commissioners appointed for Improving the Sanitary Condition of Barracks and Hospitals.
——— of Commissioners appointed to inquire into the best mode of Distributing the Sewage of Towns.
——— of Commissioners of Sewers of the City of London.
Sanitary Review.

INDEX.

W. TROUNCE, PRINTER, CURSITOR-STREET, CHANCERY-LANE, LONDON.

www.ingramcontent.com/pod-product-compliance
Lightning Source LLC
Chambersburg PA
CBHW020543270326
41927CB00006B/699

* 9 7 8 3 3 3 7 1 2 6 4 6 9 *